EFFECTIVENESS OF FOOT REFLEXOLOGY VS HOT FOOTBATH ON PREMENSTRUAL SYNDROME AND DEPRESSION AMONG ADOLESCENT GIRLS

CINU ABDEESSO

TABLE OF CONTENTS

CHAPTER I
INTRODUCTION

1.1 Background of the study

The word adolescence comes from 'adoloscere' a Latin word which means 'to come to maturity'. It is a period of spectacular growth and development. In this period a change over takes place from childhood to adulthood and is a very imperative and sensitive period of one's life. This transition from childhood to adulthood involves dramatic physical, sexual, psychological and social developmental changes and it poses risks to their health and wellbeing. (WHO, 2018).Adolescents require special attention and protection.(UNICEF,2019).The sudden and rapid physical changes that adolescents go through make them very self conscious.Girls may be anxious if they are not ready for the beginning of their menstrual periods.(Medline plus,2017).

According to the World Health Organization's expert committee (WHO,2018) adolescence is defined as the period in human growth and development that occurs after childhood and before adulthood, from ages 10 to19 and account for more than 1/5thof the world's population. There are about 350 million adolescents comprising about 22% of the population in the countries of South East Asia region. Biological processes constrain many aspects of this growth and development, with the onset of puberty marking the passage from childhood to adolescence. It is a time period of life with special health and developmental needs and rights. It is also a time to acquire knowledge and skills, learn to manage feelings, emotions and relations, and acquire attributes and abilities.

India has the largest population of adolescents in the world. 20% of people in our country encompass adolescents.(UN report, 2014).As per the report of the sub-group on adolescents for the 10th five year plan, they comprises one fifth of the world's population and have been on growing trend. According to the planning commission's population projections (2011) in India they account for 21% of the population. According to American Academy of Paediatrics (AAP, 2012) adolescent period is generally divided into three stages: early adolescence, normally ages eleven to fourteen; middle adolescence, ages fifteen to seventeen; and late adolescence, ages eighteen to twenty-one. Various developmental tasks mainly physiological growth,intellectual, psychological, social and developmental tasks are merged into these years.

Adolescent girls are one of the vulnerable groups in the society. The sudden and rapid physical changes that adolescents go through make them very self-conscious, sensitive and worried about their own body changes. They may compare themselves with their peers. Because physical changes may not occur in a smooth, regular schedule, adolescents may go through embarrassed stages, both about their look and physical harmonization. Girls may be apprehensive if they are not ready for the beginning of their menstrual periods. If adolescents appear to be secluded from their peers, uninterested in school or social activities, or doing poorly at school, work, or sports they need to be evaluated. (Cromer, 2011). Adolescents rely on their families, communities, schools, health services and their workplaces to find out a wide range of important skills that can help them to cope with the pressures they face and make the transition from childhood to adulthood fruitfully.

Onset of menarche is one of the most important changes occurring during adolescent period. The response to menstruation depends upon awareness and knowledge about the subject. Although menstruation is a natural process, it is connected with several misconceptions and practices, which result into adverse health outcomes. In various parts of India, there are several cultural traditions, myths and misconceptions related to menstruation, which make them vulnerable to reproductive health problems.There is very little cognisanceabout menstruation among girls when they first experience it. Social prohibitions and negative attitude of parents in discussing the related issues has obstructed the access of adolescent girls to right kind of information.

Jagruti Prajapati (2015) conducted a study to assess the knowledge and the practices of menstrual hygiene among 155 adolescent girls in GMERS Medical College, Gandhinagar, Gujarat. The result shows only 39.8% girls know about menstruation before menarche. Similarly Lahme, et al. (2018) in their study on factors impacting menstrual hygiene and their implications for health promotion among adolescent girls (13-20 years) menstruation and menstrual hygiene was inadequate. Additionally Sultan,etal. (2017) conducted study among 350 school girls between 10-18years of age at Bhopal stated that majority of the girls had limited knowledge of facts on menstruation and the need of adolescent girls to have accurate and up to date information about menstruation and its proper management and healthy menstrual practices. As adolescent girls have poor knowledge on reproductive health it is essential to give them adequate information about this. Hence the researcher decided to empower adolescent girls about premenstrual syndrome and its management through foot reflexology and hot foot bath technique as they are a promising group to the country's development.

Menstrual Problems

A woman plays a pivot role in the family and is a guiding factor behind all achievement and strength of the family. If she is not healthy the whole family condition becomes miserable. Menstruation is a normal physiologic process for all women. It is a universal event during a woman's life and around 90% women perceive one or more symptoms during the days before menstruation. Menstrual irregularity includes absent, infrequent, heavy, prolonged, or painful periods. It occurs in 14% to 25% of women of childbearing age. (National Institute of Child Health and Development, 2017).

Menstrual disorders are a prevailing problem in adolescents. These disorders are often the cause of concern for the patients and their families. Thecommonmenstrualdisordersinadolescent girls are dysmenorrhea, premenstrual syndrome (PMS), menorrhagia, metrorrhagia, amenorrhea, hypomenorrheaand oligomenorrhea (Trihealth, 2017).It is estimated that 15% of adolescent girls pursue medical help at least once during periods, but probably many more do not present because of shame. Menstrual irregularity has been reported in 55–82% of adolescents in the first 2 years post menarche, decreasing to 20% after around 4-5 years (Pillai, O'Brien andHill, 2009). Anandha Lakshmi, et al. (2011) investigated problems related to menstruation among adolescent girls and revealed that the prevalence of dysmenorrhea was 51% and that of the pre-menstrual syndrome was 67%. As premenstrual syndrome is a major problem disturbing a large number of female adolescent populations the researcher decided to focus on premenstrual syndrome among adolescent girls for the study.

Premenstrual Syndrome (PMS)

Premenstrual syndrome (PMS) is a major clinical problem distressing a large number of women populations. It refers to a group of physical and psychological symptoms occurring during the luteal phase (7-14 days prior to menstruation) of menstrual cycle and relieved by the onset of menstruation. The diagnostic definition for PMS established by the American College of Obstetricians and Gynaecologists states that a woman's symptoms must be present in the 5 days before her period for at least three menstrual cycles in a row, end within 4 days after her period starts and interfere with some of her normal activities (ACOG, 2015).

A woman who experiences mood symptoms is likely to experience these symptoms steadily and predictably, whereas physical symptoms may come and go. Symptoms may get worse as menstruation approaches and subside at the beginning or after several days of menstruation. (Adele Pillitteri, 2010). The complaints includes emotional instability, anxiety, irritability, depression, abdominal pain, breast tenderness, fatigue and changes in appetite. Each woman who experience PMS symptoms will be fairly predictable and constant but may be dissimilar from other women.

PMS prevalence and impact

The National Women's Health Information Center (2011) reported that due to PMS 30-40% women suffer with some impairment in daily activities, 75% women have some symptoms of PMS and severe PMS is reported by 3-8 % women. In many adolescents these symptoms may generate severe undesirable consequences and may harm the complete physical health

of a woman as well as interpersonal relationships, daily routine, and work productivity. It may affect their families and their social relationships, including low self-esteem, low tolerance to stress and feelings of inadequacy. (Tenkir Addis, Fisseha Nebreed & Ayele Biniyam, 2009).

Table 1.1 International and National prevalence rate of PMS

Country	Prevalence %	State	Prevalence %
US	90	Mumbai	75.7
UK	95	Chandigarh	79.4
Brazil	87.5	New Delhi	63
Nigeria	36.1	Gujarat	42-58
Japan	64.6	Madhya pradesh	60.5

Malaysia	74.6	Tamilnadu	55.3
Iran	98.2	Mangalore	13.33
China	30.4	Sri Lanka	65.7
Spain	73.7	Kerala	45.8

According to Royal College of Obstetricians and Gynaecologists (RCOG, 2008) 75% of women experience symptoms of PMS and 5% have severe symptoms such as depression, anxiety, irritability and breast tenderness which severely disrupts their everyday life. Fikru Wakjira Tolossa and Mebratu Legesse Bekele (2014) investigated the prevalence of PMS fromthe sample size of 258 adolescent girls aged 18 to 25 years, found that 144(83.2%) had at least one PMS symptoms during their menstrual period. The prevalence rate of PMS according to DSM-IV was 37%. Among them about 49(28.3%) were missing the classes, around 17(9.8%) students were missing exams, 14 (8.1%) were getting low grade scoring and 3(1.7%) reported

withdrawal from their learning. 83(48%) were seeking medical treatment for PMS. Among them 63(36.4%) were using pain killers, 13(7.5%) participants were used hot drinks like coffee and tea and 7(4%) were using exercise and massage therapy.

Various studies conducted on PMS revealed that these symptoms are more common and severe among high level educated women. Studies conducted in community, the prevalence of PMS was found between 5.9% and 90% in women in the age group of 15–49. Kamat, Nimbalkar, and Nimbalkar (2012) conducted a cross sectional study in India on PMS and found that the prevalence of moderate to severe PMS was 17.3% and PMDD was 4.7%. 95% girls had at least one PMS symptom, 68.8% had at least one moderate to severe PMS symptom, 49.9% had one or more physical symptoms and 89.8% had more than one PMS symptom. 37.1% had disruption of daily activities while 24.2% had absenteeism from school/college due to PMS. 75.4% girls felt that PMS was a normal part of menstruation and 50% reported moderate to severe stress. 21.4% had physical symptoms every menstrual cycle.

Rizk, Mosallam, Alyan and Nagalker (2010) reported that PMS had a significant negative impact on quality of life of adolescent girls which interferes the school performance, social interactions, life style and emotional well being. A study conducted on frequency, intensity and impact of PMS among medical students in Isra University hospital, Hyderabad by Nisar, Zehra Haider, Munir and Sohoo (2008) found that 59.5% had mild PMS, 29.2% had moderate and 11.2% had severe PMS.Biruk Kelbessa, et al. (2017) stated that a total of 51.94% of the respondents had symptoms with mild severity and 32.72% reported moderatePMS symptoms, while 15.55%

with severe PMS symptoms and interfere their daily activities like school performance and interpersonal relationships. Among the respondents 59.3% not utilized any of coping method, 20.93% used change in diet, 15.11% used medication and 4.65% used exercise as coping mechanism.

Delara, Borzuei and Montazeri (2013) investigated the prevalence and associated factors of PMS in 1379 adolescent school girls aged between 14 and 19 years at Iran reported that 99.5% of the students had at least one premenstrual symptom. Among these, 66.3% was mild, 31.4% moderate and 2.3% severe. Of these 814 girls 59% met the diagnostic criteria for premenstrual dysphoric disorder. Most often reported symptoms were back pain, lethargy, fatigue and anxiety. Dinnerstain, Lehert, Backstrome and Heinnman (2010) stated that both physical and psychological symptoms of PMS have significant impact on quality of life of adolescent girls. Later so many studies conducted on PMS and revealed it is related to high suicide and accident rates, employment and social absentee rates, poor academic performance and acute psychiatric problems. (Martina Bertello, 2014).

Causes of PMS

The exact cause of PMS has not been identified. It may be associated with social, cultural, biological, and psychological factors. Changes in neuronal hormones (progesterone on the neurotransmitters serotonin and gamma-amino butyric acid) play a major role in the cause of PMS, but this has not been proven. PMS appears more in women who are obese, who perform lessexercise and are of lower academic achievement.High caffeineintake,deficiency of certain vitamins (B6 and D) and minerals(magnesium, manganese and zinc) and stress may precipitate PMS.

Symptoms

There are more than 200 premenstrual symptoms were recognized over the past years, which incorporate three main factors: mood disorders, pain and discomfort, and bloating. Mental symptoms include: confusion, difficulty concentrating, or forgetfulness, fatigue and feeling slow or sluggish, feelings of sadness or hopelessness, feelings of tension, anxiety, or edginess, irritable, hostile, or aggressive behaviour, with outbursts of anger toward self or others, loss of sex drive, mood swings, poor judgement, poor self-image, feelings of guilt, or increased fears, sleep problems (sleeping too much or too little). The most common physical symptoms include: bloating or feeling gaseous, back pain, weight gain, swelling of extremities, water retention, nausea, muscle and joint pain, breast tenderness, clumsiness, constipation or diarrhoea, food cravings, headache, less tolerance for noises and lights, abdominal pain. (National Association for PMS, 2014).

Diagnosis

In order to identify and confirm the diagnosis of premenstrual syndrome women can maintain a prospective record of her PMS symptoms on a premenstrual symptom diary or a symptom calendar for at least two menstrual cycles. (Julia Craner, Mayo Foundation for Medical Education and Research, 2012). This will help to establish if the symptoms are limited to the premenstrual time and are recurring. Many standardized instruments have been developed to describe PMS, including the Calendar of Premenstrual syndrome Experiences (COPE),the Prospective Recordof the Impact and Severity of Menstruation (PRISM), and the Visual Analogue Scales (VAS).The prospective symptom record must maintain over a 1 to 2month period. Any calendar used for this purpose must obtain information on areas such as

symptoms, severity, and timing in relation to the menstrual cycle, and baseline level of symptoms in the follicular phase. (Robert, Reid, Allison and Case, 2015).

Treatment for PMS

The initial management for PMS is in general self-help techniques like healthy nutrition, dietary supplements, increased exercise and stress reduction (Anna Rushton, 2010; Reproductive Psychiatry Resource and information centre, 2010; Jean Hailes foundation for women's health, 2009). In case of mild to moderate PMS symptoms and the symptoms which lasts for less than one week these measures can be emphasized. The National Health Service dietary changes to alleviate PMS include eating a healthy, balanced diet, eating small meals, limit consumption of salty foods, drink plenty of water, get plenty of sleep 7 to 8 hours, eat lots of compound carbohydrates, eat calcium rich foods,consume vit E, vitamin B6, magnesium, manganese rich foods and avoid caffeine and alcohol, regular exercise, reducing stress, take painkillers such as ibuprofen or paracetamol to ease the pain, keep a diary of your symptoms for at least 2 to 3 menstrual cycles (NHS, 2018).

Association of Women's Health, Obstetric and Neonatal Nurses (AWHONN) suggest 150 minutes of moderate physical activity or 75 minutes of increased intensity activity/week will help in relieving stress and PMS and it overall improves the well-being of an individual.Non-steroidal anti-inflammatory drugs (e.g. ibuprofen)have been used to treat pain.Aspirin,ibuprofen, and other NSAIDs may be given for headache, backache, menstrual cramping, and breast tenderness.

Jarvis, Lynch and Morin (2008) evaluated the use of pharmacologic and non-pharmacologic treatment for PMS and PMDD symptoms and data were obtained through searches of MEDLINE and OVID and reported that life style modifications and exercise are first line management for symptoms of PMS. Complementary and alternative medicine has been evaluated for use in PMS/PMDD and has produced conflicting results. Although many complementary and alternative therapies for PMS are not evidence based, it is generally agreed among health professionals treating women with PMS that an integrated approach is beneficial for the majority of women.

Foot reflexology

Reflexology is an entirely natural treatment whose aim is to normalize and harmonize the functions of the body. Reflexology is one of the most effective complimentary therapies in which application of pressure to specific points on the feet breaks up crystalline deposits of uric acid, calcium and lactic acid and clears blockages and releases toxins in those areas results in stress reduction, and causes a physiological change in the body. (Maine Council of Reflexologists, 2015).The Reflexology Association of Canada (2017) defines "Reflexology is a natural healing art based on the principle that there are reflexes in the feet, hands, and ears, which represent every part, gland, and organ of the body". While applying pressure on these reflexes, reflexology relieves tension, improves circulation, and helps promote the natural function of the related areas of the body. Reflexology, or zone therapy, is a therapeutic method of relievingpain by stimulating predefinedpressure points on the feet and hands.This controlled pressure allays source ofthe discomfort. In the absence of any particular malady or abnormality, and it is also promoting good health and for preventing illness as it may be for relieving symptoms of stress, injury, and illness. By doing this touching therapy, any part of the body that is the sourceof pain, illness, or potential debility can be enhanced through the application of pressure at the respective foot or hand location.

Denise Tiran (2010) wrote that there is a growing body of evidence to demonstrate touch and therapies involving manual contact as a pain-relieving strategy, since touch impulses reach the brain before pain impulses and the impact on endorphin release aids this. It has also been demonstrated that anxiety and cortisol levels may be reduced, specifically with reflexology. Massaging or pressing each area can stimulate the flow of energy, blood, nutrients, and nerve impulses to the corresponding body zone and thereby alleviate ailments in that zone. (Stephen Barrett, 2015).

One of the theories regarding foot reflexology massage is that, since 75% of the human health problems are caused by psychological pressures and tensions and there are more than 7000 nerves in each foot, feet massage and stimulating their nerves reduce tension and create relaxation, and as a result of this body maintains the equilibrium. Chinese people believes that massage improves life energy through releasing serotonin and melatonin neural interface, as a result of this body feels less fatigue and result in improvement of depression and sleep. (Mardasi, Najar, Haghighizadeh, 2013). Since so many years reflexology massage is used as a useful method in various countries suchas China, Egypt, and India. Various research studies shows that massage therapy is an ancient therapy, which results in major improvement in anxiety and muscle pain, and it should be performed by an experienced therapist is a safe and sound method (Cutshall, et al. 2010).

According to Piran Zarifian (2017) the benefits of reflexology are: it relieves pains and aches, stimulate nerve function, makes feet healthier, promotes relaxation and better sleep, relieves premenstrual syndrome and menopausal symptoms, lowers blood pressure, relieves cancer symptoms and detoxify the body from toxins, improve blood circulation, boost metabolism and improve brain power.

PMS and Foot reflexology

Various studies on reflexology shows it is effective in many health problems including gynaecological conditions. According to Reflexology Association of Canada, (2017), reflexology technique is effective in complaints allied to menstruation like dysmenorrhoea, amenorrhea, premenstrual syndromes and menopausal problems. Other benefits of reflexology are, it provide relaxation and stress reduction, improve circulation in lymphatic and cardiovascular systems, helps the body to normalize naturally without adverse side effects and providing preventative health care.

According to American Medical Association (AMA) more than 85% of the illnesses are due to nervous stress and tension. Research has proved that PMS is a psycho physiological and a stress induced disorder and that stress is the main reason for the symptoms of PMS (Gollenberg, 2010). The proponents of reflexology claim that this technique stimulates nerves, increase
blood supply, reduce stress, maintain wellness and promote better health and general well being of the individual. Foot reflexology is a successful means of stress reduction and it is expected to relieve premenstrual symptoms.

Hot foot bath

Hot foot bath therapy is a form of hydrotherapy. It is the external or internal usage of water in any of its forms (water, ice, steam) for health promotion or treatment of varied diseases with various temperatures, pressure, duration, and site. It is one of the naturopathic treatment method used extensively in ancient cultures including India, Egypt, China, etc. (Flemingand Gutknecht, 2010). A hot foot bath is a local immersion bath covering the feet and ankles at temperatures ranging from 100° to 115° F (43°C-46°C) for 10-30 minutes (Joe and Elsa Willis, 2009). It aid to draw blood from the inflamed and congested body part. When we immerse the feet in hot water the congested blood which is present in the distant parts of the body flows to the dilated blood vessels in the legs and feet. Various areas of the body such as brain, lungs, abdominal and pelvic organ congestions can be relieved by hot foot bath technique.

Hydrotherapy acts on the healing properties of its thermal and/or mechanical effects. It is acting by the body's reaction to the pressure exerted by the water, to hot and cold stimuli, to the sensation of the water itself, to the protracted application of heat. Nerves help the sensation of the skin deeper into the body which in turn stimulates the immune system, improving circulation and digestion. It also influences the production of stress hormones, and decreases the body's sensitivity to pain and encouraging the flow of blood. The heat aid in soothing and making the body quiet, and to slow down the activity of internal organs. When an individual is experiencing anxiety or tense muscles, heat is recommended in the shower or bath. For stressed out and tired feeling, warm shower or bath followed by a short cold shower to help stimulate the body and mind is recommended. Pain or stress may lead to chemical changes in the body that may result in increased pulse rate and

blood pressure. Regular hydrotherapy treatments help in reducing these symptoms by relieving and relaxing the swollen joints and slowdown the process of stress reaction.

This helps the body to calm down and relaxed and helps to reduce the pain. (Pramod **Kerkar, 2018).**

Effects of hot foot bath

While doing hot foot bath the heat initially causes dilation of the blood vessels of the feet and improve circulation. Five minutes after the treatment stasis of the blood in the feet develops, which draws the blood away from the other congested areas of the body. Hot foot bath therapy also increases metabolism of the body and increases the body temperature. Mechanism of foot bath is that soaking foot in warm water stimulates sense of touch and reduces sympathetic activity and reduced sympathetic nerve activity is the main mechanism of increased comfort and reduced pain in patients. (Mardasi, Najar and Haghighizadeh, 2013).Warm foot bath may increase peripheral blood flow and peripheral temperature and due to heat loss without increasing core body temperature, improves falling asleep and sleep quality. Studies show that soaking feet in warm water is more effective than taking a bath in terms of facilitating falling asleep and increasing sleep quality. (Liao, Chiu and Landis, 2008).

Hot foot bath is beneficial in the following health problems: neuralgia, ovarian and menstrual problems, indigestion, asthma, pneumonia and influenza, cold hands, bladder, kidney, throat and ear inflammations, high blood pressure and any condition requires detoxification. When giving hot foot bath therapy the blood in the feet and under legs gets heated, which leads to opening of the pores of the skin and starts to sweat and thus removes toxins

from the body, improves circulation and causes strengthening of abdominal and reproductive organs,helps to normalizes the menstrual cycle and relieves tensions of the heart, beneficial in the case of common cold and in the first stage of fever, gives relief from painful feet and rheumatism, useful in managing chill, fatigue, nosebleed, plantar warts, and pulmonary congestion,

it boosts the immune system and increases lymph flow. (Yamamoto, Aso, Nagata, Kasugai and Maeda, 2011).

1.2 NEED FOR THE STUDY

Good health is the happiest thing in a human life. The most significant and sensitive period in the life cycle of a human being is the adolescent period.Various physical, emotional and social changes are taking place in an adolescent period due to the hormonal influences. In India adolescents constitutes around 243 million. (UNICEF, 2018).Adolescent girls constitute a vulnerable group and mainly in India the female children are neglected one. Menstruation is still considered as something unclean or dirty in Indian society. The reaction of adolescent girls to menstruation depends upon awareness and knowledge about it. In India, nearly one-fourth (27.7%) of the female population falls in the 15-29 years age-group. This age is a transition or change over phase of life associated with spurt of physical, mental, emotional, and social development. (Raval, et al. 2016).Rapid health changes are taking place in adolescents. It is the shared responsibility of the health care stakeholders, health care professionals, families and communities at global, national and local levels to construct the adolescents with optimum health and development.

Wong (2011) investigated attitudes towards menstruation and pre-menstrual syndrome among Turkish women found that the participants had

more negative attitudes towards menstruation. He had also reported that nearly 5-95% participants were suffering from at least one PMS symptoms. Studies show an estimated three of every four menstruating women experience some form of PMS. Due to varying pressures around school, work, families, relationships, social media, and the incessant series of transitions involved in simply being an adolescent, teens today are under more stress than ever before. (Sara Villanueva, 2015).

Menstrual cycle is a normal monthly function, but the menstrual related problems are most common among adolescent girls and have an undesirable outcome on their performance in academic and other activities of daily life which may lead to school absenteeism during menstrual days. (Noorbakhsh Mahvash, et al. (2012).It is relevant to mention here that in one year alone in India, 5,857 children, or more than 16 children per day, committed suicide because of failure in examinations (National Crime Records Bureau & Ministry of Home Affairs, 2008). PMS affect educational performance and emotional well-being (Nisar, 2008; Nagalker, 2010). Lifetime psychiatric illness also common among adolescent girls with premenstrual syndrome (Heinemann, 2010).

Raval, Panchal, Tiwari, Vala, &Bhatt (2016) investigated the prevalence of PMS among 529 college students at Gujarat found that the prevalence of PMS was 18.4%. Moderate to severe PMS was 14.7%. The symptoms commonly reported were fatigue/lack of energy, decrease interest in work, and anger/irritability. The most common functional impairment item was school/work efficiency and productivity. Deevra Norling (2015) in her article she had mentioned that apart from the physical and emotional misery it inflicts, premenstrual syndrome impact badly on interpersonal relationships,

productivity and absenteeism in the workplace. More than 150 PMS symptoms a woman can manifest during this period, some of it are irritability, mood swings, backache, headaches, breast tenderness; bloating, fatigue and even depression occurs during PMS.

In India, the prevalence of PMS found in 10-19 years old girls has been reported to be greater than 50%. (Sharma, Malhotra, Taneja, &Saha, 2010).Many studies suggest that premenstrual discomfortand dysmenorrhea are the main reason of frequent short term school absenteeism among adolescent girls and it reduces the productivity of the adolescents. Currently adolescent girls are using medications to relieve menstrual pain mainly the drugs inhibiting prostaglandin synthesis such as non-steroidal anti-inflammatory drugs. Various reports show these drugs carry their own side effects.

Buddhabunyakan, et al. (2017) investigated the prevalence of PMS among 399 high school students aged 15-18 years at Thailand found that 248 participants (85.8%) reported having at least one of the symptoms of PMS. The three most common somatic symptoms were breast tenderness (74.4%), headache (70.9%), and abdominal bloating (46.5%). The three most affective symptoms were angry outbursts (97.7%), anxiety (73.3%), and irritability (68.6%). In most cases these symptoms were rated as mild to moderate in severity.

The effect of alternative and complimentary therapy on pain reduction is less apparent. Many of the Indian studies could not be traced by the investigator in this area which might be due to lack of clear data from Indian women regarding the important aspects of women's life. This necessitates an in depth investigation and assessment of PMS. Hence the

researcher felt the need to find the prevalence of premenstrual syndrome symptoms and other premenstrual discomforts among adolescent girls and the role of foot reflexology and hot foot bath in reduction of these symptoms. Reflexology and hot foot bath studies provide information to the people to lead healthier, happier, and more productive lives. Studies show that people who are using reflexology and hot foot bath therapy consequently likely to be healthier. These studies open doors to reflexology and hot foot bath therapy being used in combination with other health care approaches.

A study conducted by Sareh Abdollahi Fard, Mahrokh Dolatian, Reza Heshmat and Alavi Hamid Majd (2012) to determine the effect of foot reflexology on PMS among 90 adolescent girls in Iran. Result revealed that 25.12% mental symptoms and 19.34% physical symptoms were relieved after receiving foot reflexology. Similarly Padmavathi

(2015) in her study conducted in Erode had reported that reflexology is an effective intervention to reduce the level of premenstrual syndrome among adolescent girls.

Sujan,Rao,Kisan, Abhishekh,Nalini,Raju and Sathyaprabha(2016) stated in their study regarding the influence of hydrotherapy on clinical and cardiac autonomic function in migraine patients significantly reduced the frequency and intensity of headaches after the treatment. Similarly Arshpreet Kaur and Naveen Kumar (2017) conducted a study on the effectiveness of hot foot bath on sleep. 15 minutes of warm foot bath was administered for experimental group. The findings of the study revealed that warm foot bath helps in improving sleep onset time and reducing insomnia.

The review of literature concerning PMS and CAM therapies has highlighted a number of areas of interest. It is evident that PMS of a chronic

nature is a common and distressing problem, which is most suitably viewed within a psychosocial perspective. In addition, although there are a variety of treatments available for the management of the condition, few have been shown beyond doubt to be effective. Contemporaneously there has been a rise in the use of CAM therapies, with PMS being one of the most common consulting conditions. Thus it is suggested that an increasing number of sufferers are seeking alternative solutions in the form of CAM to manage the condition, usually at considerable financial cost.

Thus the aim of the current investigation was to address the distinct lack of research in this area and present the controlled trial of reflexology in the context of PMS. Furthermore, in order to explore the notion that relaxation experienced during treatment is the mechanism of action in reflexology, hot foot bath and was used as a comparison condition in the current study.

1.3 SIGNIFICANCE OF THE STUDY

Future of our nation lies in the hands of our youth. In order to achieve this the youth must be physically and mentally healthy. When the body is stress free and unwavering, it can cope with the everyday stresses and strains of life much more efficiently andeffectively. A study conducted by Joshi, et al. (2010) stated that in India prevalence of premenstrual syndrome is 38.3%. According to study done by Dennerstein, et al. (2010) on the effect of premenstrual syndrome on activities of daily life reported that premenstrual symptoms had negative effects on activities of daily life and their incomelevel. They concluded that both physical and mental premenstrual symptoms have significant impact on quality of life.

21

Severe PMS symptoms have negative impact on academic and social performances of the students. Investigator felt that teaching reflexology technique and hot foot bath therapy in relieving PMS symptoms and associated symptoms of depression will help in coping with the negative impacts of PMS among the adolescent girls. Students are the promising group to country's development. Therefore the investigator felt a strong need to take up this study to assess the prevalence of PMS among adolescent girls and the
effect of alternative and complimentary therapies in relieving premenstrual syndrome symptoms and associated symptoms of depression.

Reflexology and hot foot bath are non-invasive safe therapy for preventive health, curative and complete well being. This study will provide information regarding the technique of foot reflexology and hot foot bath and its effect on reduction of premenstrual syndrome symptoms. This study will aid to develop skill in providing efficient reflexology treatment and hot foot bath therapy for effective management of premenstrual disorders. Survey of 170 reflexology studies from 21 countries shows that reflexology is effective and imparting a variety of physical and psychological concerns (Patricia Lavelle, 2010). This study will emphasis among learners on knowledge about the special features of foot reflexology and hot foot bath such as this treatment is safe and simple. It is economical and compatible, free from side effects, it gives permanent heal and also can use as a preventive treatment. It also will help to know various alternative management and effective utilization of research based practice.

It is well approved that foot reflexology therapy effectively facilitates blood and lymph circulation which accelerate the excretion of waste, soften, and stabilize the movement of muscle, joints, and tendons, reinforce muscle

strength, and promote relaxation. (Lee, Han, Chung, Kim and Choi, 2011).Various studies shows chronic health conditions seem to respond well to reflexology and hot foot bath. Among the reflexology studies conducted in China, over 300 studies report says reflexology technique provides improvement in wide variety of health conditions. A survey conducted at Denmark showed that 21.4% Danish population had used reflexology and have experienced relief from various discomforts.In 2007 a survey conducted at Norway showed 5.7% Norwegian population used reflexology to reduce pain and other discomforts within 12 months. (Dee Braun, 2009).

Hydrotherapy is most commonly understood to mean the treatment of illness through the use of water with the objective of ridding the body of toxins that may be inflicting joint pain and inflammation. Water healing is one of the oldest, safest and cheapest methods of treatment and can be used to relieve the symptoms of arthritis, anxiety, back pain, cellulitis, muscle weakness, premenstrual syndrome, stress, troubled sleep and fibromyalgia. Hydrotherapy works by using water motion to stimulate the touch receptors on the skin, thus relieving tight muscles and releasing naturally occurring chemicals called endorphins. Water is healing, refreshing, relaxing, soothing and comforting; this also boosts blood circulation and promotes general well being.

Various studies have conducted on PMS in the West and a very little number of research studies have been conducted in Asia. During the student period and while working in the college, the investigator had come across students being continually becoming absent during menstruation and also felt that very high mood variations and other negative symptoms which affects the scholastic and individual life among them which could also be

attributed to PMS. During professional life investigator felt that PMS have an impact on workplace, which leads to reduction in performance efficiency among colleagues and students.Severe PMS symptoms have negative impact on academic and social performances of the students. Reflexology and hot foot bath are non-invasive, cost effective and a technique with application of hand; it can be well implemented by a skilled nurse. Due to high prevalence and high loses resulted from PMS among the employees and students and due to reduction of the abilities of adolescents and selecting safer treatment alternatives, the researcher decided to compare the efficacy of this technique with hot foot bath on reducing the intensity and duration of PMS.

1.4 STATEMENT OF THE PROBLEM

A study to compare the effectiveness of Foot reflexology vs Hotfoot bath on premenstrual syndrome and depression among adolescent girls at selected educational institutions in Pathanamthitta district, Kerala, India.

1.5 OBJECTIVES

Objectives of the study are to

- Determine the prevalence of premenstrual syndrome and depression among adolescent girls

- ❖ Determine the effectiveness of foot reflexology on premenstrual syndrome and depression
- ❖ Determine the effectiveness of hot foot bath on premenstrual syndrome and depression

- ❖ Compare the effect of foot reflexology on premenstrual syndrome and depression with control group.
- ❖ Compare the effect of hot foot bath therapy on premenstrual syndrome and depression with control group.
- ❖ Compare the effect of foot reflexology vs. hot foot bath on premenstrual syndrome and depression
- ❖ Find the association between selected demographic variables with post premenstrual syndrome and depression. (age, BMI, place of residence,age at menarche, class performance, class missing during menstruation, menstrual duration, menstrual interval, menstrual flow)

1.6 RESEARCH HYPOTHESIS

H_1: There is a significant difference in premenstrual syndrome among adolescent girls who receive foot reflexology than who do not

H_2: There is a significant difference in depression among adolescent girls who receive foot reflexology than who do not

H_3: There is a significant difference in premenstrual syndrome among adolescent girls who receive hot foot bath therapy than who do not

H_4: There is a significant difference in depression among adolescent girls who receive hot foot bath therapy than who do not

H_5: There is a significant difference in premenstrual syndrome among adolescent girls who receive hot foot bath therapy than who receive foot reflexology

H_6: There is a significant difference in depression among adolescent girls who receive hot foot bath therapy than who receive foot reflexology

1.7 OPERATIONAL DEFINITIONS

Effectiveness

An art of estimating the outcome of alternative /complementarytherapies like foot reflexology and hot foot bath techniques rendered to adolescent girls on reducing the level of premenstrual syndrome and depression. The pre and post test scores were obtained using the standardized Moos Menstrual Distress Questionnaire (Rudolf Moos, 1969) for measuring premenstrual syndrome and Institute for Personality and Ability Testing (IPAT) questionnaire for depression (Samuel Krug and James Laughlin in 1976)to measure the level of depression.

Foot Reflexology

Involves the physical act of applying pressure to the feet with specific thumb, finger and hand without the use of oil or lotion to reduce the premenstrual symptoms and depression. A total of six groups with 10 adolescent girls in each group were grouped for the session. Foot reflexology was given by the researcher once in a week, 15 minutes for 3 months.

Hot foot bath

Involves the immersion of feet and ankles to hot water of temperature ranging from 100-115°F to reduce the premenstrual symptoms and depression. A total of six groups with 10 adolescent girls in each group were grouped for the session. Hot foot bath was given by the researcher once in a week, 15 minutes for 3 months.

Premenstrual syndrome (PMS)

Premenstrual syndrome (PMS) refers to a group of physical and psychological symptomsoccurring during the luteal phase of menstrual cycle and relieved by the onset of menstruation. The symptoms include both physical symptoms such as breast tenderness, abdominal pain and bloating, abdominal cramps, head ache, changes in appetite, nausea, vomiting, and fatigue. Psychological symptoms such as depression, anxiety and unrest. These symptoms may be related to hormonal and emotional disorders.

Depression

Depression is a state of mind which is characterized by a negative sense of inadequacy and lack of activity. It is a mental state in which the person affected experiences feelings of gloom and downturn in mood, which may be relatively transitory and may be due to something complex. The most common behaviour includes feelings of sadness, despair, low self-esteem, low self-reproach and discouragement. In specific to the study this could be experienced by the adolescent girls during the luteal phase. It is measured using the standardized IPAT Questionnaire for depression.

Adolescent girls

Girls in the age group of 17-19 years studying in 1st and 2nd year bachelor degree classes in selected arts and science colleges of Pathanamthitta district and has been identified to have premenstrual syndrome and depression as detected using Moos Menstrual Distress Questionnaire and IPAT Questionnaire for depression.

27

1.8 ASSUMPTIONS

- Troublesome symptoms need management
- Relaxation promotes healthy behaviour
- Early detection of premenstrual syndrome promotes mental health
- A relaxed mind influences the perception of events.
- Nurse investigator may develop relationship with the adolescents to implement intervention
- Adolescents will provide honest answers to the survey questions.

1.9 DELIMITATIONS

- PMS and depression were measured only by verbal report of the samples instead of any objective measurements
- The study is delimited to adolescent girls at selected arts and science colleges in Pathanamthitta district

The study is delimited to the adolescent girls with premenstrual syndrome and depression only

CHAPTER II
REVIEW OF LITERATURE

Literature review refers to an intensive, extensive and systematic examination of publications relevant to the research study. It is an essential step in the development of research project. It helps to develop insight into the subject and directs the researcher to develop the plan.

2.1 RELATED LITERATURE

The literature pertaining to the study entitled **"the effectiveness of foot reflexology vs hot foot bath on premenstrual syndrome and depression among adolescent girls"** is reviewed under the following headings.

2.1.1 Knowledge on menstrual health and problems among adolescent girls
2.1.2 Prevalence and impact of premenstrual syndrome
2.1.3 Depression experienced among adolescent girls with PMS
2.1.4 Research related to foot reflexology on PMS
2.1.5Research related to hot foot bath on PMS symptoms

2.2 CONCEPTUAL FRAMEWORK

Conceptual framework used for the study was Modified conceptual framework based on Nola .J. Pender's health promotion model (2006).

2.1.1KNOWLEDGE ON MENSTRUAL HEALTH AND PROBLEMS

Late adolescents or emerging adult hood population is growing fast in India and almost 66 million populations belong to adolescent girls. It is one of the crucial periods in the life and is a bridge between child hoods to adulthood. Emerging adulthood actually an increased risk taking period. Adolescents often lack knowledge on reproductive health including menstruation which can be due to socio-cultural barriers in which they grow up. Our society is having misconception regarding sex and sex education. Thus the parents are reluctant to talk to their children about these matters. Hence majority of adolescents do not have access to information and education on sexuality, reproduction, sexual and reproductive health and rights and even they do not have access to preventive and curative services. The adolescents are facing so many issues in the society due to this ignorance.

The adolescent girls are affected with health related problems due to bad hygiene related practices concerned to menstruation. The event of menarche may be associated with taboos and myths existing in some traditional society have a negative impact for women's health, particularly their menstrual hygiene. Attitude of parents and society in discussing the menstrual and sexual issues are barriers to the right kind of information, especially in the rural areas. There is very less knowledge and many misconceptions about menstruation among adolescents in India before and even after the menarche. This usually leads to undue fear, anxiety, and undesirable practices.

In most of the cultures menstruation is considered as a matter of embarrassment. Many of the adolescent girls usually have lack of scientific

knowledge and menstrual hygienic practice during menstruation and puberty, also adolescent girls often are hesitant to discuss this embracing topic with their health care-providers and often hesitate to pursue help in regard to the menstrual problem from external sources. The reaction to menstruation depends upon the awareness and knowledge about the subject. The way in which a girl learns about menstruation and its associated changes may have an impact on her response to the event of menarche. If we pay little attention for these groups we can lessen the risk of potentially harmful outcome from sexual behaviour such as fear and stigma of menstruation. Therefore, girls should be educated about menstruation and healthy menstrual practice.

Yadav,Joshi,Poudel and Pandeya (2018) a cross sectional study was conducted to assess the current knowledge, attitude and practice of school adolescents on menstrual hygiene management in Doti district in far-western Nepal. Their sample included 276 students from grade seven and eight from 11schools. Self-administered structured questionnaire was used for data collection. Results showed that 26.4% samples had good knowledge and 67.4% samples had fair knowledge on menstrual hygiene practices. Around 50% samples had positive attitude towards menstrual hygiene management. They concluded that attitude and practices on menstrual hygiene among school girls need to improve.

A cross-sectional study was conducted by **Shoor (2017)** to study the knowledge and attitude towards menstruation, practices of menstrual hygiene, enumerate the common menstrual morbidities and to elicit the health-seeking behaviour regarding menstrual health among adolescent girls.They had selected 452 girls from six schools and onepre university college aged between 10-19 years from Maralur, Tumkur by purposive sampling and

used a semi-structured, pretested questionnaire for data collection. The results revealed that only 37.39% girls were aware about the importance of menstrual hygiene, 34.1% girls had the right perception about menstruation, 35.32% of girls reported their fear during first time when attained menarche and 11.08% girls said they had no restrictions during menstruation. They concluded that the school girls had less than satisfactory knowledge on menstruation, but following good practices regarding menstrual health.

Shubha Srivastava and Madhuri Chandra (2017) conducted a study on the knowledge of school girls regarding menstrual and reproductive health and their perceptions about family life education program at Gandhi medical college, Bhopal. The study was conducted in five schools and 537 girls participated in the study. A questionnaire was given to the school girls to know their knowledge, attitude and perception regarding menstruation, reproduction, nutrition and their views on the quality and usefulness of the family life skills sessions. Results revealed that the source of information of the girls were their mothers.Most of them were considering menstruation is shameful and young girls face many restrictions. They reported knowledge regarding menstruation, reproduction, contraception and diet is still lacking among the school girls.

A cross-sectional study on knowledge, belief, practices and sources of data pertaining to menstruation and hygiene among adolescent girls of junior colleges, Kuppam, Andhra Pradesh, India was done by **Aruna Marati Savanthe and Vrushabhendra Halevoor Nanjundappa (2016)**. Study samples included were 1,160 college-going adolescent girls aged 15–19 years. A pretested questionnaire used for data collection.The study results

revealed that the mean age at menarche was 13.83 years. 24.7% samples were aware about menstruation before menarche, 48% reported dysmenorrhea. They concluded that the knowledge regarding safe and clean practices on menstrual hygiene was needed in adolescent girls to ensure a healthy reproductive life.

Shriram Vitthal Gosavi, et al. (2015) did a community based cross-sectional study to determine the awareness and practices about menstrual hygiene and its impact among migrant adolescent girls of Dera, the corporation area of Nashik, Maharashtra. Purposive sampling method was adopted for selection of samples. A semi-structured schedule with open ended questions was used for data collection process and in-depth interviews conducted among the selected girls. Results revealed that 75% girls were not aware about menarche and they reported that the myths and misconceptions about menstrual practices are still continued.

Reda Ibrahim, El-Mowafy, Maha Moussa, Mohamed Moussa and Hanan Hassan El-Ezaby(2014) studied aboutthe effect of health education program on knowledge and practices about menstrual hygiene among adolescent girls at orphanage homes in Damietta City, Egypt. Total sample of 234 adolescent girls aged between 14-16 years were selected for the study. The study revealed that adolescents lacked appropriate knowledge and practicesabout menstruation in the pre-program phase. After implementation of the program considerable improvements were noticed in adolescents' girls' knowledge and practice. Therefore they concluded that the educational program was successful in attaining its aim of positively changing the knowledge and practice of menstrual hygiene.

Rupali Patle and Sanjay Kubde(2014)carried out a community based cross sectional study on menstrual hygiene in rural and urban adolescent girls at Indira Gandhi government medical college, Nagpur. 310 adolescent girls in the age group of 10-19 years from each area were the participants. Girls were interviewed by house to house survey.Their knowledge and attitude regarding menstruation as well as hygienic practices during menstruation was assessed.The study concluded that the awareness regarding menstruation was more in urban adolescent girls (63.38%) as compared to rural (47.57%). The study results also revealed that 62.03% of urban girls were using commercially available sanitary pads as compared to 43.4% of rural girls.

An epidemiologic study conducted by **Kamath, Ghosh, Lena and Chandrasekaran(2013)** to explore the knowledge and practices regarding menstrual hygiene among rural and urban adolescent girls in Udupi Taluk, Manipal, India. They had selected 270 urban girls and 280 girls from rural area aged between 13-16 years through random sampling technique. Result showed that around 34% participants were aware of menstruation prior to menarche, and mothers were the main source of information among both groups.70.4% of adolescent girls were using sanitary napkins as menstrual absorbent, and 25.6% were using both cloth and sanitary napkins. They concluded that there is a need to equip the adolescent girls with knowledge regarding safe and hygienic practices to enable them to lead a healthy reproductive life.

A descriptive cross sectional study on knowledge and practices about menstrual hygiene among higher secondary school girls at Varanasi district revealed that menstrual hygiene is one of the very important risk

factor for reproductive tract infections and it is a vital aspect of the health education to the adolescent girls. 120 adolescent girls were participated in the study. Results showed that about half of the girls (58.3%) were aware about menstruation prior to attainment of menarche. The mean age of menarche was found to be 12.98years (+0.77).The most common menstrual pattern was 3 days/ month. Mother was the first informant regarding menstruation in case of 41.66%girls.85.8% girls believed it as a physiological process. Regarding practices, only 50.8% girls informed about the use of sanitary pads during menstruation. Most of the girls 49.16% used old plain cloth as menstrual absorbent. About 82.5% girls practised different restrictions during menstruation. **(Pragya Verma,Ahmad&Srivastava, 2013)**

Jarrah and Kamel (2012) conducted a descriptive cross sectional study to investigate the attitude and menstruation-related practices in Jordanian school-aged girls; and identify the influence of premenstrual preparation on girls' attitude and menstruation-related practices. Data were collected from 490 school girls aged between 12-18 years from different districts of Jordan. They have used Menstrual Attitude Questionnaire and Menstrual Practices Questionnaires for collecting the data. Study results showed that poor attitude toward menstruation and low menstrual practices were significantly associated with inadequate premenstrual preparation. In their study conclusion reported a need to prepare girls for menstruation before menarche and the role of schools and teachers as health educators to provide sexual education and menstrual health to the adolescent girls.

A descriptive, cross-sectional study by **Ray Sudeshna and Dasgupta Aparajita (2012)** on determinants of menstrual hygiene among 190 adolescent girls aged between 13-19 years of a rural secondary school of

Hoogly district, West Bengal. They used a self-administered pre-tested structured closed-ended questionnaire for interview. Results revealed that 42% girls were aware about menstruation prior to attainment of menarche. The study concluded that adoption of high quality menstrual hygiene will play an important role in prevention of reproductive tract infections. Therefore promoting knowledge and positive attitudes towards management of menstruation and related problems among the adolescent girls are necessary to reduce the potential risk of infections.

A community based cross sectional study was conducted in urban slum area under urban health training center of Katuri medical college hospital, Guntur, Andhra Pradesh (**Keerti Jogdand &Pravin Yerpude, 2011)**regarding menstrual hygiene. Result revealed that only 36.19% girls were aware of menstruation prior to the attainment of menarche. During menstruation 34.63% girls reported use of old cloth for protection and 78.99% girls were restricted to attend religious occasions during menstruation. Study concluded that adolescents' girls need more information about menstrual health.

Sabyasachi Ray **and** SujataMaiti Choudhury **(2011)** carried out a cross-sectional study on knowledge and information on psychological, physiological and gynaecological problems among adolescent school girls in semi urban area of West Bengal, India. A total of 521 adolescent girls aged 10–19 years were selected randomly from two secondary schools. Collected all information by using open-ended pre-tested questionnaire. It was observed that 18%of the respondents had good knowledge, 60.7% had moderate or some knowledge and21.3% experienced very poor knowledge of puberty, pubertal problems and their prevention. The study concluded that knowledge

regarding sex education was poor among the adolescent girls and they suggested that the school based sex education programs are particularly good at providing information, skills development and attitude clarification.

2.1.2 STUDIES REGARDING PREVALENCE AND IMPACT OF PMS

Saadia and Faiza (2018) conducted a descriptive cross sectional study on menstrual problems among women and their effect on the work at Omdurman Military Hospital, Sudan. They have selected one hundred non-health care worker women randomly in this study. Results revealed that the age of first menstruation range between 11 and 17 years with meanage of (13.19±1.2SD).79% women had regular menstruation. Premenstrual syndrome (PMS) occurred among 7% of women and menstrual symptom occurred among 60% of them and psychological changes exist in 43%. Menstrual problems and effect on their work were found among 47% of them. 79% women manage their symptoms with alternative therapy and 36% used medical therapy while physical methods used by 45%. They concluded that
menstrual problems were very prevalent among women and it affects daily activities in work.

Arafa, Senosy, Helmy and Mohamed (2018) conducted a population based cross sectional study to investigate the prevalence and patterns of dysmenorrhea and premenstrual syndrome (PMS) among girls in Beni-Suef, Egypt. The study was conducted on 4122 girls between the age of 12-25 years. Result showed that high rates of dysmenorrhea (92%) and PMS (86.3%) were present among girls. The most commonly reported symptoms were backaches (63.3%), generalized aching (62.4%), and nervousness (43.5%) respectively.

Rumana Akbari, Sudharani, Sherin Joseph Xavier, Ramya, Nagendra Gowda and Suryakantha (2017) investigated a cross sectional study to know the prevalence of PMS and to study the factors associated with PMS among medical students of Basaveshwara medical college, Chitradurga. Self-evaluating questionnaire was used to collect data. Symptoms were analysed one week before periods, during periods and one week after periods. Result revealed that the prevalence of PMS among the study participants were 31.1%, among them 20%, 7.4% and 3.7% showed mild, moderate and severe

formrespectively. They concluded that the prevalence of premenstrual syndrome was high among college students.

Buddhabunyakan, Kaewrudee, Chongsomchai, Soontrapa, Somboonporn and Sothornwit (2017) conducted a prospective study to assess the prevalence of PMS in Thai high school students in Khon Kaen, Thailand. Premenstrual experiences according to the diagnostic criteria proposed by the American College of Obstetricians and Gynaecologists were given to the participants to prospectively complete for 90 consecutive days. Results showed that out of 289 participants 86 participants (29.8%) reported having PMS. The most common somatic symptom was breast tenderness (74.4%) and affective symptoms among participants with PMS were angry outbursts (97.7%). They reported that PMS was associated with various problems related to educational activities, including lack of concentration and motivation, poor individual work performance, poor collaborative work performance, and low scores.

Ghadeer, Shuhayb, Luwaim, Jughaiman and Haji (2016) conducted a cross sectional study to find out the prevalence of premenstrual syndrome and its impact on the daily activities of students in King Faisal

University. They have selected 354 women aged between 19-25 years and used a self reported questionnaire includes biographical data, premenstrual symptoms, and possible risk factors that may influence the physical impairment during PMS. The result revealed that 92.2% of the participants experienced moderate to severe PMS. They concluded that premenstrual syndrome is common among King Faisal University students.

Tibin Joseph, Nandini and Sabira (2016) did a non-experimental descriptive survey study to assess the prevalence of premenstrual syndrome among adolescent girls in a selected college, Thrissur. Study findings showed that out of 60 samples, 10% had PMS.Among them 75% were having mild PMS, 15% were having moderate PMS and no one was experiencing severe PMS. The common symptoms reported were 73% back ache, 65% were having tiredness and 60% were having irritability, 48% having tension, 42% having mood swings and 22% suffering from muscle stiffness, 20% having sleepingproblems 18% having dizziness, painful breast, feeling of suffocation and nausea or vomiting. They have concluded that the incidence of PMS is increasing rapidly among adolescent girls due to various factors and lifestyle changes.

Ranjana Mandal, Aditya Prasad Sarkar and Supriti Ghorai (2015)did a cross-sectional descriptive study at Kolkata city from the students of class IX to XII. Total 278 students were participated in the study. Their study results concluded that the prevalence of PMS was 54%. Out of the affective symptoms the study report showed depression was 45.7%, anger 61.2%, irritability 88.1%, anxiety 51.8%, confusion 46.4%, rejection 24.8%, breast pain 22.7%, abdominal distension 37.5%, headache 40.6% and swelling of limbs by 5% of girls.

NasimNaeimi (2015) determined the prevalence of premenstrual syndrome in students of Sistan and Baluchestan University. They have selected 201 students randomly who were living in the dormitories for their study. According to thestudy results 36.3% of the samples suffered from premenstrual dysphoric disorder and 85.6% of subjects indicated the symptoms of PMS.72.6% samples had fatigue and 62.7% samples had lethargy and abdominal pain. They concluded PMS is highly prevalent among University students.

A cross sectional study was carried out by **Hetal jain and Avani Parek (2015)** to assess the prevalence of premenstrual syndrome in married and unmarried females of 18-26 years of age from Charotar region,in Gujarat.400 samples participated in the study. Out of 200 unmarried females who participated in this study 63% had mild to moderate pemenstrual symptoms, 34.5% had moderate to severe and 2.5% had severe symptoms of PMS. Among the 200 married females 65.5% had mild to moderate premenstrual symptoms, 31.5%had moderate to severe and 3% had severe symptoms of PMS. Fatigue (60%) was the most common symptom reported by both married and unmarried women. 50% of the samples reported decrease interest in work, social activity and home activity and 50% samples reported physical symptoms such as breast tenderness, headaches, joint/muscle pain, bloating and weight gain. They concluded premenstrual symptoms were prevalent in focus group of Charotar region.

Fikru Wakjira Tolossa and Mebratu Legesse Bekele (2014) conducted a cross-sectional study among systematically selected female students of Mekelle University college of health sciences, Mekelle town, Northern Ethiopia to assess the prevalence, impacts and medical management

of PMS. They had selected a sample size of 258 students ranged from 18-25 years for the study. Results showed that among the participants, 144(83.2%) had at least one PMS symptoms with their menstrual period. The prevalence of PMS according to DSM-IV was 37%. About 49(28.3%) reported frequent class missing, 17(9.8%) exam missing, 14(8.1%) low grade scoring and 3(1.7%) of them reported withdrawal from their learning associated with their PMS. Only 83(48%) participants sought medical treatment for their

PMS. The study concluded that a high prevalence and negative impact of PMS on students of Mekelle University and academic performance impairment were significantly associated with the PMS.

Manal Ahmad Al-Batanony and Sultan Fahad AL-Nohair (2014) investigated theprevalence of premenstrual syndrome and the impact on quality of life among University medical students at Al Qassim University, KSA. They have selected unmarried medical students aged 18-25 years with regular menstrual period for the last 6 months for their study. Results showed that the prevalence of PMS among the study group was 78.5%, of them, 5.9% had severe form of PMS. They concluded that the PMS is a prevalent, but under treated, disorder among medical students in KSA, which adversely affecting their quality of life.

A study was conducted by **Ashraf Direkvand-Moghadam**, **Kourosh Sayehmiri**, **Ali Delpisheh**, **and** **Satar Kaikhavandi** **(2014)** to investigate the worldwide prevalence of PMS using meta-analysis method. After reviewing many articles they selected seventeen studies and analysed. Their result showed that from the total of 17 papers 18803 people surveyed and found out the pooled prevalence of PMS was 48%.Pooled prevalence of PMS was reported 40% in Europe, 85% in Africa, 46% in Asia and 60% in

South America. The lowest prevalence of PMS was reported in France (12%) and the highest prevalence of PMS was in Iran (98%).

Brahmbhatt, Sattigeri, Shah, Kumar and Parikh(2013) a survey was conducted among 50 young and 50 middle aged women of S.B.K.S Medical Institute and Research Centre, Vadodara, Gujarat to find the prevalence of premenstrual syndrome and its management. They used a feedback questionnaire covering various aspects related to PMS were obtained from 50 participants belonging to each group. The participants belonged to different range of literacy. It was revealed that 42% experienced PMS regularly, while 58% occasionally. Among the 100 participants 68% suffered with backache, 64% leg cramps, 62% fatigue, breast tenderness and anger whereas 58% suffered with anxiety and generalized body ache. Of all the sufferers only 34% had consulted doctor for the treatment of PMS. The study concluded that irrespective of the age,premenstrual syndrome is a common problem faced by women.

A cross sectional study conducted by **Waghachavare, Dhumale, Kadam, Quraishi, Kumbhr and Gore (2012)** on the problems related to menstruation in late adolescent girls from selected higher secondary schools and are residing in the rural area from Western Maharashtra. They selected all the willing girls for the study as samples and used pre-tested, pre-validated self-administered questionnaire to collect the data. Their study result revealed that 40.3% samples were suffering from dysmenorrhea. Weakness, giddiness, headache, excessive bleeding, and irregularmenstruation were observed as problems.32 subjects had premenstrual dysphoric disorder. They concluded that menstrual problems were present among the adolescent girls, which highlights the need for proper professional counselling.

Aruna (2012) investigated the effectiveness of cognitive behavioural nursing strategies on premenstrual syndrome among adolescent girls from Thiruvallur district, Chennai. The researcher selected 320 adolescent girls in the age group of 14-18 years from 2 government schools and two private schools using simple random sampling technique. Result showed that 643 (55.3%) adolescent girls did not have premenstrual distress. 241(20.7%) and 239 (20.4%) adolescent girls had mild and moderate level of premenstrual distress respectively. Strong premenstrual distress was found among 20(1.7%) adolescent girls. 23(1.9%) adolescent girls had severe premenstrual distress. Study concluded that premenstrual syndrome is prevalent among adolescent girls.

Obeidat, Alchalabi, Abdul-Razzak and Al-Farras (2012) conducted a cross sectional study to determine the prevalence of premenstrual symptoms among a sample of female students in one of the University in Jordan. A total of 177 female students aged between 18 to 24 years who experienced primary dysmenorrheaparticipated in the study and completed a self-administeredquestionnairetocollectinformationconcerningdemographics, menstruation-related information and associated specified premenstrual symptoms. Result showed that among the 177 participants 91.5% had two or more symptoms among which fatigue, mood swings, anxiety, abdominal bloating, and depression were the most prevalent symptoms. They concluded that premenstrual symptoms are very common in young women with primary dysmenorrhea.

Mingqi Qiao, etal. (2012) investigated the prevalence of premenstrual syndrome,frequency and severity of premenstrual syndrome symptoms and premenstrual dysphoric disorder among Chinese women of

reproductive age. They screened women aged between 18–45 years and used daily record of severity of problems questionnaire to assess the symptoms prospectively over 2 months. The study results revealed that the incidence of PMDD was 2.1% and the prevalence of PMS was 21.1%. The most common symptoms reported were irritability (91.21%), breast tenderness (77.62%), depression (68.31%), abdominal bloating (63.70%) and angry outbursts (59.62%). They concluded that premenstrual syndrome symptoms are prevalent among Chinese women.

A school based descriptive study done by **Chandraratne and Gunawardena (2011)** to determine the experience of premenstrual syndrome among a sample of Sri Lankan adolescents at Government schools of Colombo. Samples were aged between 13-16 years. The result showed that premenstrual symptoms were experienced by 65.7% of the population. Common somatic symptom was fatigue (29.9%) and affective symptom was feeling sad/hopeless (29.6%). PMS prevalence was 8.75%. Multivariate analysis reported the presence of chronic physical illness ($P = 0.001$), dysmenorrhea ($P < 0.001$), and regular menstrual cycles (P = 0.006) as correlates of PMS. Presence of PMS significantly distrupted"in school" activities, relationships and activities of daily routines (P<0.005) indicating a high negative influence on adolescents' daily life. Only 9.7% sought help from medical practitioners for their premenstrual symptoms and a majority had not perceived it as a condition to report.

Omu, Al-Marzouk, Delles and Oranye(2011) investigated a prospective observational study on the prevalence of premenstrual dysphoric disorder among non-treatment seeking female students at the college of nursing, Kuwait. This study also investigated the effects of the disorder on

their academic performance as indicated by their grade point average and rate of absenteeism at clinical training. The rate of premenstrual dysphoric disorder was 5·6%. Hypotheses tested shows no significant effect on students' academic performance but there is a significant association with absenteeism at clinical training. They concluded participants with high luteal scores believe that the condition have lowered their quality of life by making them isolated during the period.

A cross sectional nationwide survey conducted by **Dueñas, et al. (2011)** to assess the prevalence of premenstrual syndrome and premenstrual dysphoric disorder in a cohort of Spanish women aged between 15 and 49 years. Result showed that of the 2108 participants, 1554 women (73.7%) complained of some of the premenstrual symptoms during the last 12 menstrual cycles. A total of 1415 (91%) women reported isolated symptoms and 139 (8.9%) presented a moderate/severe premenstrual syndrome. They concluded that the prevalence of premenstrual symptoms (73.7%) and premenstrual dysphoric disorder (1.1%) in Spanish women aged between 15 and 49 years is similar to that reported in other Western countries.

Zohre Mahmoodi (2010) investigated the frequency and severity of premenstrual syndrome and its associated signs and symptoms. They have selected 500 undergraduate students of Iran University of medical sciences, department of nursing-midwifery and management information schools for their study. 255 students completed the premenstrual daily symptom diary forms. Their study result showed that 200 (78.43%) students were suffering from some degree of PMS. 62% samples were having mild PMS, 36% were suffering from moderate PMS, and 2% of them were having severe PMS. 24% were having severe mood symptoms and 3% of them had severe

behavioural symptoms. They reported a significant positive relationship between behavioural symptoms, physical and mood symptoms and concluded that the health professionals should recognize physical and emotional symptoms of PMS and provide them with an appropriate education and medical intervention.

An exploratory study conducted by **Petta, Osis, De Padua, Bahamondes and Makuch (2010)** to describe the perspectives and attitudes of Brazilian women toward premenstrual syndrome. They have selected 6 major cities, 1 in each geographic region of Brazil and 1 in the federal district. The study samples were women aged 18-40 years who consulted at public healthcare services or who were members of staff/faculty at University. Results showed that among 1053 women, 96.1% had heard of PMS, 65.4% considered that all or almost all women experienced the condition, 87.5% reported that symptoms occurred prior to menstruation and 60.3% were thinking that they had PMS at the time of the interview. The emotional and physical symptoms most frequently mentioned were nervousness/anxiety (76.4%), mood swings/crying (55.7%), pain, swelling, and tenderness of the breasts (37.3%) and cramps (45.4%).

Thamilselvi (2010) studied on premenstrual syndrome of adolescent girls in Cuddallore district of Tamilnadu. This study was intended to examine the type of pre-menstrual syndrome experienced by adolescent girls between the age group of 10-19 years in rural and urban areas of Cuddalore district of Tamilnadu. The sample size was 300 comprising of 158 adolescent girls from rural and 142 from urban areas respectively. About 55% suffered from premenstrual syndrome. The major syndromes included were white discharge and pains of various natures.

Dennerstein, Lehert, Keing, Palsa and Choi (2010) studied a population-based cross-sectional survey on the impact of premenstrual symptoms on activities of daily life among 1202 women aged 15-49 years, were selected by random sampling in cities of Hong Kong, Pakistan and Thailand. They used check list of 23 premenstrual symptoms, socio demographic and lifestyle variables, overall impact of premenstrual symptoms on activities of daily living (ADL). Symptoms were classified into their intensity, persistence in each cycle, and impairment of ADL. The result showed that 74% of women were not affected or minimally affected in ADL, 17% had a clinically significant effect on daily activities and 9% were severely affected in daily activities. ADL were predominantly affected by premenstrual symptom severity. They concluded that PMS occur frequently and have a significant impact on daily life for a proportion of women.

Navdeep Kaur and Ramesh Thakur (2009) conducted a descriptive study to assess the premenstrual syndrome and coping behaviour among nursing students at PGIMER, Chandigarh. 248 students from all classes were selected as samples for their study and collected data from them. Results revealed that the most common (79.43%) problem was lower abdominal pain. 66.12% having backache, 52.01% having low efficiency of work performance. Most of the students were using healthy coping strategies. 89.11% do not blame themselves for the problem, 75.4% accepted it as nothing can be done. 98% samples were taking hot or cold drinks for PMS.

Ballagh and Heyl (2008) conducted a study to assess the prevalence of PMS among the reproductive age group women. Their study result showed that 85% of reproductive aged women experience physical or emotional changes with their menstrual cycle and up to 40% of women were

bothered by menstrual cycle related symptoms such as dysmenorrhea and PMS. These condition influence women's lives, relationships, work and is the most common reason for absenteeism for women younger than the age 30.

An observational study was conducted by **Nisar, Zehar, Haider, Munir and Sohoo (2008)** to determine the frequency and severity of premenstrual symptoms in Isra University hospital, Pakistan. They had selected 172 unmarried medical students aged 18-25 years with regular menstrual period for the last6 months using convenience sampling. PMS related data were collected on daily record of severity of problems for two prospective cycles. Health-related quality of life data was collected on medical outcome study using Short Form 36. Their study result showed that ICD-10 criteria of PMS were met by 51% girls. Among them 59.5% had mild PMS, 29.2% had moderate and 11.2% had severe PMS. 5.8% samples were having PMDD. The symptoms reported were anger, irritability, anxiety, tiredness and difficult in concentration.

2.1.3 STUDIES RELATED TO PMS AND DEPRESSION

MinakshiParikh, Nimesh Parikh, and Sweta Parikh (2015) conducted a study in Western India to assess the prevalence, severity and symptom profile in adolescent girls and to assess co-morbid depression among them. They used specifically designed premenstrual assessment form based on DSM-IV as tool for data collection. Co-morbid depression was assessed using Hamilton depression rating scale. Result showed that prevalence of PMS was 12.22% with all of them showing work impairment during the affected period. 18.52% of those had co-morbid depression.

Seyed Saeed Sadr, Seyed Mehdi Samimi Ardestani, Katayoon Razjouyan, Mahboobeh Daneshvari and Ghazal Zahed(2014) conducted a cross sectional research to evaluate the association between PMS and depression in medical students. 100 female medical students of Shahid Beheshti University of medical sciences at Iran were selected as samples for their study. The study samples were divided into two groups, experimental and control after administration of demographic questionnaire and PMS questionnaire made by researchers based on diagnostic and statistical manual of mental disorders. Then, they completed Beck's depression inventory. Result showed that from 100 participants, 55% had PMS and 45% had no PMS. In the PMS group 30% had no depression; 38% had mild depression; 23% had moderate depression; and 7% had severe depression. In the group with no PMS 60% had no depression; 20% had mild depression; 17% had moderate depression and 2% had severe depression. The depression score was significantly higher in PMS group (p =0.04).Study revealed that PMS had an elevated frequency in medical students. In students with PMS, depression rate was higher than students without PMS.

Rudy Bowen, Angela Bowen, Marilyn Baetz, Jason Wagner and Roger Pierson (2011)investigated whether mood instability was higher in women with premenstrual syndrome than in a control group with no PMS. They prospectively studied mood and physical symptoms over two menstrual periods in 29 women with self-identified premenstrual syndrome and 31 women without premenstrual syndrome.They used the mean square successive difference derived from two times daily visual analogue scale ratings of mood as the measure of mood instability. Results revealed that the women with premenstrual syndrome showed more irritable and depressed mood instability than the women without premenstrual syndrome.

Miyaokay Akimoto (2011) carried out a study to assess the experience of PMS among adolescents with depressive disorders. In this study premenstrual symptoms in adolescents with depressive disorders were investigated by using the premenstrual syndrome scale. Questionnaires were administered to 65 Japanese female outpatients who had been diagnosed with a major depressive disorder and to 303 healthy women as control subjects. This study concluded that 28 adolescents (43.1%) with depressive disorder fulfilled certain items of the PMS scale. These adolescents were considered to have coexisting PMS and a depressive disorder, or to have premenstrual exacerbation of a depressive disorder. On the other hand, 18 adolescents (5.9%) in the control group were diagnosed as having PMS. Findings demonstrated that the occurrences of severe premenstrual symptoms were much higher in adolescent with depressive disorders than in healthy subjects.

Rapkin and Winer (2009)studied about the quality of life in people suffering from premenstrual symptoms and the associated problems inLos Angeles. The common symptoms associated with premenstrual syndrome reported in their study included irritability, fatigue, breast tenderness, anger, mood swings, depression and anxiety. These symptoms were occurring every month and lasts for an average of six days per month. Severe form of premenstrual syndrome was associated with disabling depressive disorder. Their study result also reported that during the reproductive years an affected woman experience around 3000 days of severe premenstrual syndrome symptoms which affects their work productivity and impairs the well being.

Gonda (2008) conducted a study among 63 mentally healthy women regarding fluctuation of psychological symptoms during luteal phase for three menstrual cycles by monitoring the prospective record of symptoms

and they used state trait anxiety inventory to assess the anxiety, zung self-rating depression scale to assess the depression during premenstrual period and concluded that there is a significant increase in psychological symptoms related to neuroticism and depression during late luteal phase.

Stephanie Collins Reed, Frances Levinand Suzette Evans (2008)did a study to assess the changes in mood, cognitive performance and appetite in the late luteal phase and follicular phases of the menstrual cycle in women with and without premenstrual dysphoric disorder. They have selected 29 normally cycling women (14 women who met DSM-IV criteria for PMDD and 15 women without PMDD). Result showed that there was a significant increase in dysphoric mood during the luteal phase in women with PMDD compared to their follicular phase and compared to control women.

2.1.4 STUDIES RELATED TO FOOT REFLEXOLOGY ON PMS

Ola Araby (2018) investigated a quasi-experimental pre-test post-test study to evaluate the effect of self-feet reflexology on relieving premenstrual syndrome. Systematic random sample of female students in first year who have premenstrual syndrome and fulfil the inclusion criteria from faculty of nursing at Benha University were the samples. They used self-administrated questionnaire and Menstrual Distress Questionnaire for the collection of data. The result revealed that there was a highly statistical significant difference in pain, autonomic reactions, general manifestations, concentration, behavioural change and negative affect after receiving foot reflexology therapy. The study reported that encouraging foot reflexology practice among the academic students reduce premenstrual syndrome and improve their well-being.

Laxmi Agnihotri (2017) conducted a pre experimental one group pre-test post-test design study on the effect of foot reflexology on dysmenorrhea among adolescent girls in a selected nursing hostel at Vijayapur. Samples were adolescent girls aged between 17-20 years, who were suffering from dysmenorrhoea and staying in the selected nursing hostel at Vijayapur. Numerical Pain Rating Scale was used for assessing pain. The result revealed that the mean pretest pain score was high (4.025) than the mean post test pain score of 2.425, which is highly significant. Findings indicated that the foot reflexology massage is highly effective on dysmenorrhoea among adolescent girls.

Marwa Mohamed, Asmaa El Bandrawy and Amir Gabr(2016) investigated the effect of foot reflexology and relaxation training in decreasing premenstrual symptoms in adolescent females. A sample of 50 volunteers, virgin females diagnosed as having premenstrual syndrome was selected from the students of faculty of physical therapy, at Cairo University, Egypt. Assessment of respiratory rate, heart rate, plasma cortisol level as well as daily symptoms report chart was carried out before and after the treatment program for all subjects in both groups A& B. Group A received foot reflexology in addition to relaxation training techniques twice a week for 8 weeks. Group B received only relaxation training techniques twice a week for
8 weeks. Result showed that a highly significant statistical decrease ($p< 0.05$) in heart rate, respiratory rate, plasma cortisol level as well as daily symptoms report score in group A,and in group B there was a statistical significant decrease ($p <0.05$) in all variables.

Padmavathi (2015) conducted a true experimental factorial design comparative study to assess the effectiveness of acupressure vs reflexology on

premenstrual syndrome among adolescent girls in selected schools at Erode, Tamilnadu. Samples were adolescent girls with premenstrual syndrome in the age group of 13-17 years and were selected from 2 high schools using multi stage random sampling. Assessment of level of premenstrual syndrome was measured by premenstrual syndrome scale. Acupressure to experimental group I and reflexology to experimental group II were given to adolescent girls on individual basis. Result showed that pretest mean premenstrual syndrome score (161.98 ± 6.63, which is 81%) and (160.61 ± 7.15, which is 80%) was less than the post test mean premenstrual syndrome score (82.48 ± 4.23, which is 41%) and (76.74 ± 5.2, which was 38%) in experimental group I and II respectively.The study concluded that acupressure and reflexology is an effective intervention to reduce the level of premenstrual syndrome and also the study result shows that reflexology was more effective than acupressure on premenstrual syndrome among adolescent girls.

Jissy Jacob (2013) investigated a quasi experimental study to assess the effectiveness of reflexology on premenstrual syndrome among adolescent girls in selected nursing colleges at Mangalore. Sample size was 30B.Scnursing students from 2 nursing colleges. Reflexology was given to experimental group students on the fourth day of their menstruation and continued for 24 days twice daily. Post test was conducted after 24 days of intervention by administering premenstrual syndrome rating scale. The result showed that the mean post test score (5.67±2.79) of premenstrual syndrome was lower than the pretest score (28.33±5.34).

Sareh Abdollahi Fard, Mahrokh Dolatian,Reza Heshmat and Alavi Hamid Majd (2013)conducted a singleblind controlled clinical trial study to assess the effect of foot reflexology on symptoms of premenstrual

syndrome in students of Jahrom University. 90 students with premenstrual syndrome were selected for the study. They were divided into experimental and control group. Severity of premenstrual syndrome was recorded in two cycles: pre intervention cycle and intervention cycle. The tools used were data gathering form, temporary diagnosis form of PMS, dialogue record form and beck depression test. The result showed that pre and post intervention in reflexology significantly led to decrease of average of mental symptoms (25.12%) and physical symptoms (19.34%).Their study revealed that, foot reflexology is effective in improvement of physical and mental symptoms of premenstrual syndrome.

A quasi-experimental clinical trial study was conducted by **Mahboubeh Valiani, Elaheh Babaei, Reza Heshmat and Zahra Zare (2010)** to compare the effects of reflexology methods and ibuprofen administration on dysmenorrhea in 80 female students aged between 18-25 years had primary dysmenorrhea with regular menstrual cycles and living in the dormitories of Isfahan University of medical sciences. One group receivedibuprofen treatment and other group undergonefoot reflexology. Ibuprofen was administered during three consecutive menstrual cycles and the reflexology was given during two consecutive menstrual cycles. Paired t-test results showed that mean pain intensity assessed by visual analogue scale had a significant difference after the intervention in each reflexology and ibuprofen groups. They concluded that both therapies were effective in reducing dysmenorrhea.

2.1.5 STUDIES RELATED TO HOT FOOT BATH THERAPY

Hot foot bath therapy is a form of hydrotherapy. It is a branch of nature cure and water is a great healing agent. The healing properties of

hydrotherapy depend on its mechanical and thermal effects. It exploits the body's reaction to hot stimuli. Many studies reported the physiological or therapeutic or combination effects of hydrotherapy on various systems of the body. Hydrotherapy uses water to bring temperature and pressure variations to the body. These changes are perceived by the body through nerve endings in the skin and muscle and result in neural reflex effects that are controlled by the brain and spinal cord. Warmth and pressure of water also reduce swelling and reduces load on painful joints, promotes muscle relaxation. Warm hydrotherapy also helps ease nervousness and headaches and soothes irritated vocal cord. It will also lessen the pain associated with abdominal and pelvic ailments like menstrual cramps, hemorrhoids, kidney disorders, intestinal disorders, gall bladder disorders, liver disorders and other systemic problems that cause internal pain. As hot foot bath therapy is having a positive effect on whole body systems and organs is expected to relieve premenstrual symptoms.

Hot water foot bath therapy causes blood vessels to dilate and results in improved blood circulation, which releases heat in the form of sweat and supply of oxygen to brain cell which helps in the excretion of toxins (Selvakumari, 2009).Various research studies showed that hot water foot therapy is an effective method in reducing many diseases. Aileen, (2018) in her study reported that hot water foot therapy is very effective therapy among patients with fever and help them for faster recovery.

Yelin Ko and Joo-Young Lee (2018) did a study to determine the effect of feet warming using bed socks on sleep quality and thermo- regulatory responses during sleep in a cool environment. They had selected six young males aged 22.7 ± 2.0 years were divided into two groups

randomly. The study group was receiving feet warming and other group was the control group. Sleep-onset latency, sleep efficiency, total sleep time, number of awakenings, wake after sleep onset, average awakening length, movement index, and fragmentation index were measuring by using a wrist actigraphy during 7 hour sleep period.Heart rate and body temperatures (skin and rectal) were monitored during the 7hour sleep. In the morning after awakening questionnaire on sleep quality was obtained. The results showed that sleep-onset latency was an average 7.5 minutes shorter, total sleep time was 32 minutes longer, the number of awakenings was 7.5 times smaller, and sleep efficiency was 7.6% higher for those having feet-warming bed socks during a 7-hour sleep than control. They concluded that sleep quality can be improved by manipulation of the foot temperature throughout sleeping.

Randomized controlled crossover trial study was conducted by **Chiu,Lin,Chiu and Chen (2017)** to examine the effect of home-based warm foot bath intervention to improve sleep in the chronic phase of traumatic brain injury. 23 adults with TBI were selected and randomized to receive first a 30-minute, 41°C warm foot bath and then a usual care, or vice versa, with each lasting 3 days and separated by a 3-day washout. Sleep efficiency, sleep onset latency, total sleep time, and wake after sleep onset were assessed by actigraphy. Result showed that the home-based warm foot bath significantly reduced sleep onset latency (difference -5.11 minutes) and wake after sleep onset (difference-2.57 minutes) compared with usual care. Study concluded that home-based warm foot bath is practical and effective in relieving post-traumatic brain injury sleep disturbances.

Suneesh,Kavitha Thangavel and Jeenath Justin Doss (2017) conducted a pre experimental one group pre-test post-test design to determine

the effectiveness of warm foot bath on sleep onset time among cancer patients with insomnia in NathLal Parekhcancerhospital at Rajkot. They had selected 30 cancer patients by purposive sampling method. The data was collected through general sleep disturbance scale.15 minutes of warm foot bath was administered for experimental group. The findings of the study revealed that warm foot bath helps in improving sleep onset time and reducing insomnia.

A randomized controlled trial study was conducted by **Joao Marcos Dias, et al. (2017)** to assess the impact of hydrotherapy on pain and muscle function in older women with knee osteoarthritis. Their samples included seventy three women aged 65 and above were randomized to study group (36 samples) and control group (37 samples). The study group samples received hydrotherapy in a heated pool twice weekly for six weeks and given an educational protocol. The control group received the educational protocol only. WOMAC osteoarthritis questionnaire was used to assess the pain intensity and isokinetic dynamo-meter was used for assessing knee extensor and knee flexor muscle performance. The result revealed that the hydrotherapy group had better outcomes for pain and better performance for knee flexor and extensor strength, knee flexor power, and knee extensor endurance. They had concluded that hydrotherapy is an effective method in reducing pain and improving muscle function.

Haghayeghi et al. (2016) conducted a quasi-experimental study with pre-test post-test design to investigate the effect of eight weeks of hydrotherapy on life quality and depression in elderly women over 50 years at Jahrom city in Iran. They have selected 15 elderly women over 50 years by convenient sampling. The levels of depression and life quality were measured before and after the implementation using Beck depression inventory and the

questionnaire of life quality (SF36). Hydrotherapy was given for 8 weeks (24 sessions).The result revealed that a significant difference between mental and physical aspects of life quality before and after the intervention (p-value=0.001&0.002). T test results show that there is a significant difference between the depression level of elderly women before and after the intervention of hydrotherapy exercise (p-value=0.004).

Mehdi Naseri, Ali Rahmani, Batool Nerir, Mehdi Salari,and Maryam Moshni Farahani(2016) did a quasi experimental comparative study on the effect of foot reflexology massage and foot bath on the sleep quality of patients with acute coronary syndrome. Group A received foot reflexology massage and solar plexus rotating massage for 10 minutes. Group B received foot bath in 40°C water for 10 minutes. Group C not received any intervention. Patients in the study groups were under intervention for 2 nights from the 2nd night of hospitalization and sleep quality was assessed through Verran and Snyder-Halpern subjective sleep quality questionnaire before and after the intervention. Results showed that there was no significant statistical difference among the 3 groups regarding sleep disturbance and supplementary sleep after interventions ($P>0.05$), but there was a significant statistical difference between the groups and at different timing in regard to the effectiveness after intervention.

Haylaa Nageeb, Ragaa Ali Mohamed and Hadayat Amasha (2015) estimated the prevalence of premenstrual syndrome among adolescent girls and to identify complementary and alternative therapy used by nursing schools students to minimize premenstrual syndrome using exploratory design. 1120 nursing students from all secondary technical nursing schools in Dakahlia governorate was selected as samples by purposive sampling. Interview questionnaire and modified menstrual distress questionnaire was

used for data collection. Results of the study showed that, the prevalence of premenstrual syndrome was 73.4%. Among them 87% samples were using complementary and alternative therapy to minimize premenstrual syndrome. The main complementary and alternative therapy used was herbal therapy followed by hydrotherapy, food change, massage and exercise.

Leila Valizadeh**(2015)** conducted a controlled single-blinded parallel trial clinical study comparing the effects of reflexology and foot bath on sleep quality in the elderly in Tabriz city, Iran.They used the Pittsburgh sleep quality index (PSQI) for data collection. Both experimental groups had reflexology and foot bath interventions for 6 weeks. The reflexology intervention was done in the mornings, once a week for 10 minutes on each foot. The samples in the foot bath group were asked to soak their feet in 41°C to 42°C water one hour before sleeping. Samples in the control group received no intervention.The results showed that the Pittsburgh sleep quality index scores after intervention compared to before in the reflexology and foot bath groups were statistically significant and the control group did not show a statistically significant difference.

Myeong Heui Ahn**,** So Hyun Jeon **and** Yeongmin Yoon **(2013)** investigated the utilization of stone therapy and hydrotherapy in premenstrual syndrome. Unmarried women aged 20-40 and diagnosed to have premenstrual syndrome, who wereresiding in the metropolitan area were their samples and divided into three groups as group A, B and

C. Group A received stone therapy and group B had undergone hydrotherapy. Both of stone therapy and hydrotherapy were offered to the experimental group C. Menstrual pain was assessed by using visual analogue scale. Modified menstrual distress questionnaire were used to test premenstrual syndrome. The result revealed

that, there was a significant decrease in the menstrual pain of all three experimental groups. Significant reductions in psychological and physical symptoms were observed in all three groups.

Levona Johnson (2011) conducted a quasi-experimental, single group pretest post test design study to assess the effect of hydrotherapy on the pain levels and stress levels in patients with rheumatic disease at Groote Schuur hospital, department of physiotherapy at the hydrotherapy pool in observatory, Western Cape. A sample of 19 patients of any age and racial group diagnosed with a rheumatic disease were selected as samples for the study using convenient sampling and used visual analogue scale for pain and weekly stress inventory-short form questionnaire for assessing stress level. Hydrotherapy was given once per week for 6 months. The result revealed that the mean pain score for the samples were 7.2 (SD=1.8) and a range of 4-10. Post intervention, the mean pain score was 3.7 (SD=2.2) and the range was 0-7.5. Similarly the mean event score for the participants was 7.63 (SD=6.06) and a range of 0-19.Post intervention, the mean event score was 9.4 (SD=5.9) and the range was 1-25. The study concluded that the hydrotherapy had a significant impact on pain reduction.

Yang, Chen, Lee, Fang and Chao (2010) did a study on the effects of warm-water foot bath on relieving fatigue and insomnia of the gynecologic cancer patients on chemotherapy. Experimental group samples soaked their feet in 41°C to 42°C warm water for 20 minutes every evening, starting from the evening of receiving the first chemotherapy and the participants in the comparison group did not do so. Results revealed that participants in the experimental group reported a significant reduction in fatigue and improvement in sleep quality from the second session of chemotherapy and continued to improve during the study period.

2.2 CONCEPTUAL FRAMEWORK

A conceptual framework or model is interrelated concept or abstractions assembled together in a rational scheme by virtue of their relevance to a common theme. The conceptual framework selected for this study was based on revised Nola J Pender's health promotion model 2006. Health promotion is one of the primary objectives in modern nursing. Health promoting behaviors can edge to a patient's overall sense of well-being as well as protection from disease and chronic illnesses. Pender's health promotion theory offers a holistic view of the patient, assessing the patients' background and self-perceptions. The health promotion theory can ideally be applied to all populations but is mainly important in the adolescent population since they are at a critical time and it is a transitional period in their life for making independent health care decisions.

Pender defined health as not just being free of diseaseand it also includes measures taken to promote better health and includes the patient's view of themselves and their lifestyle (Peterson & Bredow, 2009). Pender's model meant to be a "guide for exploration of the complex biopsychosocial processes that motivate individuals to engage in behaviours directed toward the enhancement of health" (Pender, 1996). Pender created this model to be "applicable to any health behaviour in which threat is not proposed as a major source of motivation for the behaviour" (Pender, 1996). Pender states that "Health is the actualization of inherent and acquired human potential through goal-directed behaviour, competent self-care, and satisfying relationships with others while adjustments are made as needed to maintain structural integrity and harmonial relationship with relevant environments"(Pender,2006).Pender also offers a classification of behaviouralexplanation of health which includes affects, attitudes, activities, aspirations and accomplishments. Her definition not only offers a holistic view of the individual but also it focus on their illness (Peterson & Bredow, 2009).

Pender's model identifies many relationships between concepts. Health promoting behaviour is described as the ultimate outcome of the model. Personal factors are independent variables that directly influence behaviour-specific cognitions and also directly effect the specific health promoting behaviour. Perceptions of self and influences on the individual directly effect dedication to a plan of action which then leads to the health promoting behaviour. Health promoting behaviours are also both indirectly and directly influenced by prior related behaviours, and directly influenced by intermediate challenging demands. Pender outlines specific assumptions in her model are based on which overall emphasize the fact that the patient has an active role in their health behaviour. It is pretended that a patient can self-reflect, actively pursue to regulate behaviour, and initiate behaviours that modify their environment. Another assumption is that health professionals apply an interpersonal influence on an individual all through their life (Pender, 1996).

Nola J Pender's Health promotion model describes three key concepts: they are individual characteristics or experiences, behaviour specific cognitions and affect and behaviour outcomes. Health promoted behaviour is directed towards attaining positive health outcomes for the adolescent girls. The health promotion model (HPM) proposed by Nola J Pender in 1982 and revised in 1996. According to this modelhealth is defined as "a positive dynamic state not merely the absence of disease". Health promotion is aimed at increasing a client's level of well-being. The health

promotion model explains the multi-dimensional nature of persons as they interact within their environment to seek health. The model illustrates the multifaceted nature of persons interrelating to their environment in pursuit of health. A thorough appraisal of this theory denotes that this model can be useful in the adolescent population but may need to be adapted in various ways to be successful. It can also be concluded that much more studies need to be done applying this model to the adolescent population.

The Health promotion model integrates nursing and behavioural science perspectives to describe the "multidimensional nature of persons interacting with their interpersonal and physical environments as they pursue health" (Pender, Murdaugh & Parsons, 2006). This theoretical framework examines the complex processes that drive an individual to participate in health behaviours. The model describes the basic factors that influence health behaviour. The central focus of the model is on eight beliefs that can be evaluated by the nurse. These beliefs are critical points for nursing intervention. Using the model and working collaboratively with the Patient/client, the nurse can help the client in changing behaviours to attain a healthy lifestyle.

Key concepts in nursing defined as a basis for the Health promotion model

Person is a bio psychosocial organism that is partially shaped by the environment but also seeks to construct an environment in which inherent and acquired human potential can be fully expressed. Thus, the relationship between person and environment is reciprocal. Individual characteristics as well as life experiences mould behaviours including health behaviours.

Environment is the social, cultural and physical conditions in which the life course unfolds. The environment can be manipulated by the individual to create a positive context of cues and facilitators for health-augmenting behaviours.

Nursingis collaboration withindividuals, families, and communitiesto generate the most.

Health in relation to the individual is defined as the actualization of inherent and acquired human potential through goal-directed behaviour, competent self-care, and satisfying relationships with others, while adjustments are made as needed to maintain structural integrity and harmony with pertinent environments. Health is an evolving life experience.

Illnesses are distinct events throughout the life span of either short (acute) or long (chronic) duration that can hinder or facilitate one's continuing quest for health.The model highlights on following three areas:

- Individual characteristics and experiences
- Behaviour-specific cognitions and affect
- Behavioural outcomes

These components lead to a logical advancement of the concepts needed to improve health and health behaviours and support. Bennett, Perry and Lawrence (2009) believe that health behaviours must be in control of the patient and mean something to the patient to be effective. Pender's model is based on two theories of human behaviour: expectancy value theory and social cognitive theory. The expectancy value theory states, "People are more

likely to work toward goals that are of value to them" (Reed & Shearer, 2009). Social cognitive theory is self-efficacy which is the confidence a person has in the ability to be successful in a task or deal. Pender's model gives guidance to assessing the patient as to readiness to learn, barriers to adherence and learning, interpersonal influences, benefits to health promotion and situational influences. All these components support the success of promoting and encouraging health behaviour change. Pender's model of degree of abstractness is a definite strength, allowing for the concepts developed for this said project to be utilized in other medical condition settings.

The health promotion model describes that each person has unique personal characteristics and experiences that affect successive actions. The set of variables for behavioural specific knowledge and affect have important motivational implications. These variables can be modified through nursing actions. Health promoting behaviour is the expected behavioural outcome and is the end point in the health promotion model. Health promoting behaviours should result in enhanced health, improved functional ability and best quality of life at all stages of development. The final behavioural demand is also determined by the immediate competing demand and preferences, which can derail an intended health promoting actions.

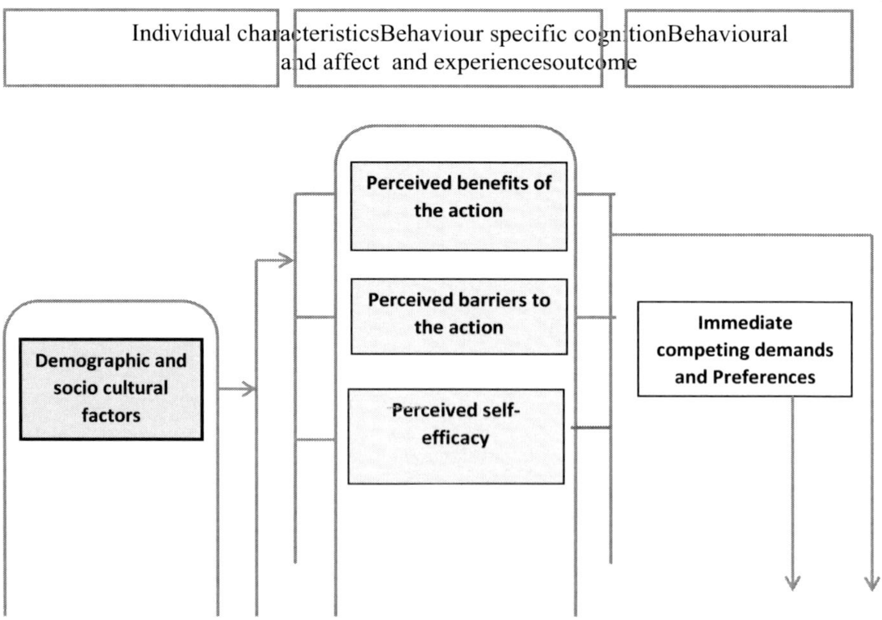

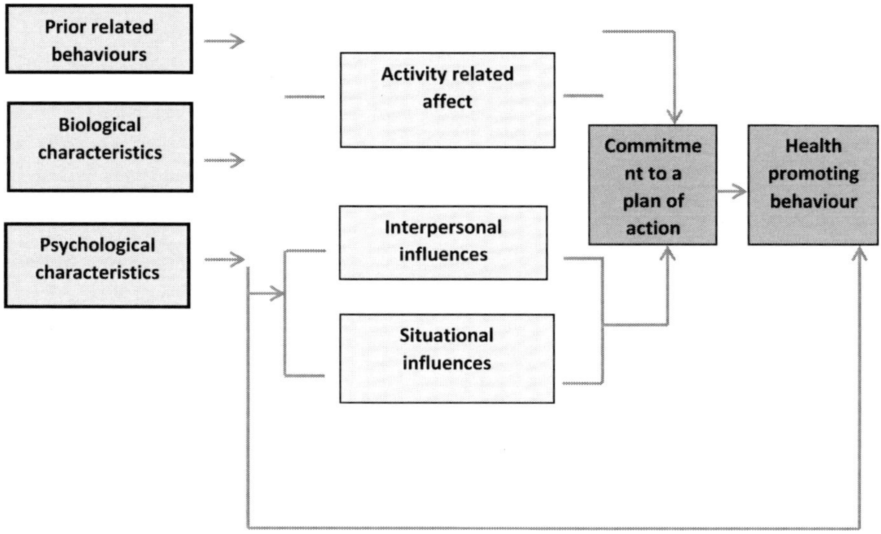

Figure 2.2.1: Nola.J. Pender's Revised Health Promotion Model (2006)

Theoretical propositions of the Health promotion model

- Prior behaviour and inherited and acquired characteristics influence beliefs, affect, and enactment of health-promoting behaviour.
- Persons commit to engaging in behaviours from which they anticipate deriving personally valued benefits.
- Perceived barriers can constrain commitment to action, a mediator of behaviour as well as actual behaviour.
- Perceived competence or self-efficacy to execute a given behaviour increases the likelihood of commitment to action and actual performance of the behaviour.

- Greater perceived self-efficacy results in fewer perceived barriers to specific health behaviour.
- Positive affect toward a behaviour results in greater perceived self-efficacy, which can in turn, result in increased positive affect.
- When positive emotions or affect are associated with behaviour, the probability of commitment and action is increased.
- Persons are more likely to commit to and engage in health-promoting behaviours when significant others model the behaviour, expect the behaviour to occur, and provide assistance and support to enable the behaviour.
- Families, peers, and health care providers are important sources of interpersonal influence that can increase or decrease commitment to and engagement in health-promoting behaviour.
- Situational influences in the external environment can increase or decrease commitment to or participation in health-promoting behaviour.
- The greater the commitments to a specific plan of action, the more likely health-promoting behaviours are to be maintained over time.

- Commitment to a plan of action is less likely to result in the desired behaviour when competing demands over which persons have little control require immediate attention.
- Commitment to a plan of action is less likely to result in the desired behaviour when other actions are more attractive and thus preferred over the target behaviour.
- Persons can modify cognitions, affect, and the interpersonal and physical environment to create incentives for health actions.

Major Concepts and Definitions

A. Individual characteristics and experience

Prior related behaviour: frequency of the same behaviour in the past. It has a direct and indirect effect on the likelihood of engaging in health promoting behaviours.

Personal factors: personal factors categorized as biological, psychological and socio-cultural. These are general characteristics of the individual which influence health behaviour. They are age, personality structure, race, ethnicity and socio economic status.

Personal biological factors: which include variables such as age, gender, body mass index,pubertal status,aerobic capacity,strength, agility, or balance.

Personal psychological factors: it includes variables such as self esteem, self-motivation, personal competence, perceived health status and definition of health.

Personal socio-cultural factors: which include variables such as race, ethnicity, acculturation, education and socio economic status.

B.Behaviour - Specific Cognitions and Affect

Perceived benefits of action: anticipated positive outcomes which will occur from health behaviour. It is the perception of the positive or reinforcing consequences of undertaking health behaviour.

Perceived barriers to action: anticipated, imagined or real blocks and personal costs of understanding a given behaviour

Perceived self-efficacy: judgement of personal capability to organize and execute a health-promoting behaviour. Perceived self-efficacy influences perceived barriers to action. So higher efficacy leads to lowered perceptions of barriers to the performance of the behaviour.

Activity related affect:it is the subjective positive or negative feeling that occurs before, during and following behaviour based on the stimulus properties of the behaviour itself. Activity-related affect which influences perceived self-efficacy that means the more positive the subjective feeling, the greater the feeling of efficacy. In turn, increased feelings of efficacy helps in generating further positive affect.

Interpersonal influences:these are cognition concerning behaviour, beliefs, or attitudes of the others. Interpersonal influences include: norms (expectations of significant others), social support (instrumental and emotional encouragement) and modelling (vicarious learning through observation of others engaged in a particular behaviour).Primary sources of interpersonal influences consist of families, peers, and healthcare providers.

Situational influences: personal perceptions and cognitions of any given situation or context which facilitates or impede behaviour. Situational influences may directly or indirectly influences on health behaviour.

C. Behavioural Outcome

Commitment to plan of action: it means the concept of intention and identification of a planned strategy leads to implementation of health behaviour.

Immediate competing demands and preferences: competing demands are those alternative behaviours over which individuals have low control because there are environmental contingencies such as work or family care responsibilities. Competing preferences are alternative behaviour over which individuals apply relatively high control, such as choice of ice cream or apple for a snack.

Health promoting behaviour: endpoint or action outcome aimed toward attaining positive health outcome such as optimal well-being, personal fulfilment, and productive living.

CONCEPTUAL FRAME WORK FOR THE STUDY

Health promotion model (HPM) was developed to explain health promoting behaviours; it can also be used for health protecting behaviours (Pender, 2006).It describes new phenomena and reveals relationship between existing phenomena. The researcher selected the Pender's health promotion model as the framework for this study because it is an empowering, holistic and competence based model and it logically integrates the multiple factors influencing foot reflexology and hot foot bath. In HPM there is a parallel between health promoting behaviours and health protecting behaviours. The revised Pender's health promotion model has been modified to provide a

better framework for the study in order to better understand the phenomenarelated to individual experience and management strategies of adolescent girls with premenstrual syndrome.Reasons for selection of health promotion model for this study were two fold. Complementary and alternative modalities of treatment is a health promotion activity and the concepts and the relationships of the health promotion model have solid experimental representation and have been found to be predictive of health promoting behaviour.

Based on Pender's health promotion model, this study emphasizes the fact that health-care professionals need to understand and address modifiable behaviour-specific variables. The study recommends that an effective empowerment strategy would be to use activity-related affect, as well as interpersonal and situational influences, as a means of facilitating and enhancing clients' health-promoting behaviours.Based on Pender's health promotion model the existing premenstrual symptoms and depression have been assessed by the investigator and the use of health promotive behaviour has been gauged with direction from HPM. The study focused on health promotion by relieving premenstrual syndrome and depression through foot reflexology and hot foot bath technique. Within the study physical and psychological symptoms during premenstrual period were the statistically significant variables.

In this study the health promotion model consists of three dimensions. These are the individual characteristics and experiences, behaviour specific cognitions and affect and behavioural outcome. The basic concepts of this study which incorporates some of the basic concepts of the health promotionmodel where individual characteristics and experience are

based on the priorrelated behaviour and personal, biological, psychological and socio culturalfactors. Behaviour specific cognitions and affect refers to the anticipated positive consequences and real blocks occur while undertaking a health promoting behaviour. It also incorporates the personal capability to execute a health promoting behaviour. Behaviour specific cognitions are affected by interpersonal and situational influences. Activity related affect explains the subjective positive and negative feeling that occurs before, during and following health promoting behaviour.

Individual Characteristics and Experiences

In this study the individual characteristics and experiences are the prior related behaviour of the adolescent girls such as prior assessment of the premenstrual syndrome symptoms and depression and the personal factors such as awareness of foot reflexology and hot foot bath. The premenstrual symptoms are very important aspects of health which disrupts the physical, psychological and social functioning (premenstrual syndrome sub scale such as pain, impaired concentration, behavioural change, autonomic reaction, water retention, negative effect, arousal and control).The researcher should first find out the presence of these signs and symptoms to identify the adolescent girls with PMS and depression. Premenstrual symptoms and depression level can be vary from mild to severe which may highly disrupt their daily activities and functions. The researcher selected adolescent girls for this study because they are more prone to affect the PMS and depression due to high educational demand from the parents, more educational activities and due to peer pressure.

The PMS and depression could be attributed due to various personal domains such as demographic variables, personal variables and gynecological

variables which influence the adolescent girls' views and response to the individual experiences. In this study the researcher identifies the level of PMS as mild, moderate, strong and severe in adolescent girls through daily symptom diary and MOOS Menstrual distress questionnaire. The level of depression as mild, moderate or severe is measured by using IPAT questionnaire for depression. MOOS menstrual distress questionnaire is using to find outthe retrospective PMS and daily symptom diary for prospective PMS. The adolescent girls who had severe PMS and severe depression will be excluding from the study. Such girls are referred to Muthoot hospital Pathanamthitta for further management. Before selecting the samples for experimental and control group an informed consent is obtaining in order to propose their willingness to participate in the study.

Behaviour Specific Cognitions and Affect

The study concentrated on behaviour specific cognitions of perceived benefits of action, perceived barriers to action, self-efficacy, activity related affect, interpersonal influences and situational influences. HPM relates individual characteristics and behaviour specific cognitions and affect to health and health behaviour. The investigator considered foot reflexology and hot foot bath knowledge as an individual characteristic that could influence health behaviour.

Perceived benefits of action are the anticipated reduction in premenstrual syndrome and depression and improvement in quality of life. Perceived barriers to action such as lack of source of information, interest, motivation and lack of knowledge on reflexology and hot foot bath affect both intention to engage in and the actual execution of health behaviours. Based on Nola J Pender's health promotion model perceived self-efficacy is the ability toperceive the PMS and depression and understand the importance of foot reflexology and hot foot bath in the management of these health problems. The participants' perception of herself efficacy is directly affected by whether she perceives the activity a positive or negative experience. The way a person perceives and understands a situation candirectly or indirectly affect health behaviour.

Activity related affect explains decrease in premenstrual symptoms and depression and increase in quality of life. Interpersonal influences such as family, peers,health care providersand support by the investigator and situational influences such as participation in the study, calm and quite environment, safe locations and reinforcement for health promotion can affect one's commitment in health promoting behaviours.

Behaviour Outcome

In this study the behavioural outcome explains, a planned strategy leads to implementation of health promoting behaviour such as relieving of PMS and depression. It is assessed by measurement of the dependent variable such as PMS and depression. The researcher assumed that the outcome of study groups would be more desirable than the control group. The girls from the control group should remain in the same level of PMS and depression.

According to the researcher the study empowered participants' to become co-planners of their care and facilitated intervention planning appropriate to participants. The conceptual framework modified for adolescent girls with premenstrual syndrome and depression was derived from Nola J Pender's revised health promotion model, which is illustrated in figure2.

Diagrammatic representation of the conceptual framework of the study

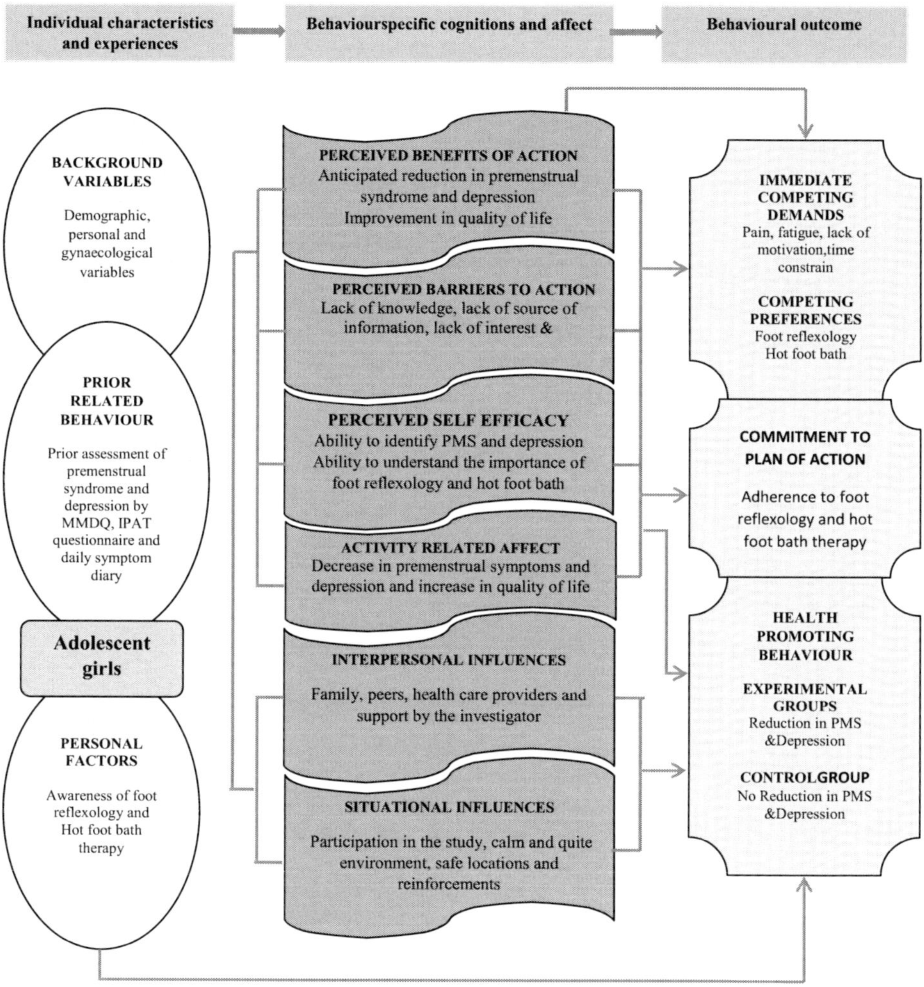

Figure 2.2.2: Modified Conceptual Framework based on Nola.J Pender's Health promotion Model, 2006

CHAPTER III
RESEARCH METHODOLOGY

This chapter deals with the methodology adopted for assessing the effectiveness of foot reflexology vs. hot foot bath on premenstrual syndrome among adolescent girls at selected arts and science colleges in Pathanamthitta district, Kerala, India. Research methodology is a way to solve the research problem, includes research approach, research design, setting of the study, variables, population, sample, sample size, sampling technique, criteria for selection of sample size and development and description of the research tool and technique, administration, scoring procedure of the tools, content validity of the tool, reliability of the tool, pilot study, data collection procedure and statistical analysis used for the study. The results of studies into the effectiveness of foot reflexology and hot foot bath for menstrual conditions such as premenstrual syndrome are inconclusive. Clinical studies of foot reflexology and hot foot bath therapy for PMS will provide evidence for practice.

3.1 RESEARCH APPROACH

Quantitative research approach was adopted for this study to accomplish the objectives of the study.

3.2 RESEARCH DESIGN

It is a true experimental study. This quantitative research used a pre-test post-test control group design with arts and science colleges as the unit of randomization. This study instituted 3 groups, 2 experimental groups

and a control group. The arts and science colleges were randomized to experimental group I, II and control group.

Table 3.2.1 SCHEMATIC REPRESENTATION OF RESEARCH DESIGN

R

Group	Pre test	Interventions	Post test
EI	O1	X1	O2
EII	O1	X2	O2
CG	O1	*	O2

R-Arts and science colleges were randomly selected

EI-Experimental group I adolescent girls who received foot reflexology

EII- Experimental group II adolescent girls who received hot foot bath

CG-Control group without any intervention

O1- Pre test assessment

O2- Post test assessment

X1-Interventions given to experimental group I in two phases.

During Phase I - checking the prevalence of premenstrual syndrome and depression by distributing MOOS menstrual distress questionnaire (MDQ), IPAT depression scale and PMS daily diary.

During Phase II - doing foot reflexology to adolescent girls by the researcher once in a week 15 minutes for 3 months.

X2-Interventions given to experimental group II in two phases.

During Phase I- checking the prevalence of premenstrual syndrome and depression by distributing MOOS menstrual distress questionnaire (MDQ), IPAT depression scale and PMS daily diary.

During Phase II –giving hot foot bath therapy to the adolescent girls by the researcher once in a week 15 minutes for 3 months.

*-Control group is asked to continue the routine measures

O2-Assessment of PMS and depression in experimental group I, II and in control group after two weeks of completing the interventions.

3.2.1 Manipulation

Interventions were implemented by the researcher to samples of the experimental groups in two phases. During phase I prevalence checking was done by distributing MOOS menstrual distress questionnaire, IPAT depression scale and PMS daily diary. During phase II foot reflexology techniques were implemented by the researcher to the experimental group I. A total of 6 groups with 10 adolescent girls in each group were grouped for foot reflexology session. This technique was performed to the adolescent girls weekly 6 days in the college hostel during evening time after the college hours. This was done once weekly 15 minutes for 3 months. Hot foot bath therapy was given by the researcher to the experimental group II. A total of 6 groups with 10 adolescent girls in each group were grouped for hot foot bath session. This therapy was given to the adolescent girls weekly 6 days in the college hostel during morning time before the college hours. This was done once weekly 15 minutes for 3 months.

Foot reflexology technique was given as an intervention for the adolescent girls in the experimental group I who were having premenstrual syndrome. The investigator does a series of procedures over the predefined pressure points on the patient's feet, by applying direct pressure using the fingers. This is to stimulate the spinal points in order to reduce pain, anxiety, depression and to improve the quality of life. The techniques used were head spin, ankle spin, ankle rotation, ankle massage, side twist, foot twist, plantar press, sole massage, sole press, dorsal press, dorsal groove press, top of foot crease slide.

Hot foot bath therapy was given as an intervention for the adolescent girls in the experimental group II who were having premenstrual syndrome. The investigator explained the procedure and checked for the contraindications. Then immersed both feet and ankles of adolescent girls in hot water (110°F) for 15 minutes, which draw blood from congested areas of the body and relieves various discomforts of the body.

The control group adolescent girls requested to continue with their normal routine and college activities and researcher completed the assessments at the same time intervals as that of the experimental groups. The control group adolescents' girls were taught the same interventions after the completion of the study.

3.2.2 Recruitment

The researcher contacted the principals of arts and science colleges of Pathanamthitta district in Kerala to take permission for conducting the research study among adolescent girls of 1st and 2nd year bachelor degree. Nine colleges were agreed to participate. Out of nine

colleges 6 colleges were selected randomly to experimental groups and control group. Researcher explained the study rationale, procedures and random allocation of colleges to the principals.

3.2.3 Randomization

Out of nine colleges agreed to participate, 6 colleges were selected randomly by simple random method to experimental groups and control group. Randomizations of colleges were accomplished by writing the names of the nine colleges on separate pieces of paper. The researcher requested one of the lecturers to pick six pieces of paper. After random selection of six colleges for the study, the researcher prepared papers with experimental group I and II or control group written upon them and requested one of the teacher to pick 2 pieces of paper and that colleges were selected for experimental group I and the same procedure were followed for selection of colleges for experimental group II and control group.

After assigning colleges to either experimental groups or control group, all female students who were studying in the 1st and 2nd year bachelor degree classes in all 6 colleges were invited to participate in the study. Out of 1168 students 1097 students showed interest in participating in the study. A detailed summary of the proposed study was explained to the adolescent girls after obtaining consent. A complete survey was done among the 1st and 2nd year bachelor degree students to identify adolescent girls who fulfilled the inclusion criteria.

Preliminary assessment was done to assess premenstrual syndrome and depression. After the first preliminary retrospective assessment, adolescent girls were requested to maintain premenstrual daily

symptoms diary for prospective record of symptoms. The researcher described the daily symptom diary. Adolescent girls were instructed to record the symptoms for one menstrual cycle in the evening. Once in a week the researcher reminded the adolescent girls about keeping the daily symptom diary. Forty days after the first visit, the same adolescent girls were asked to complete a baseline assessment using the completed daily symptom dairy. Thus, the baseline assessment included the data of two consecutive menstrual cycles.These retrospective and prospective cross sectional data were used to identity adolescent girls with mild, moderate, or strong premenstrualsyndrome and mild or moderate depression. Based on this preliminary assessment the adolescent girls who had (1) severe premenstrual syndrome as measured by MMDQ or no premenstrual syndrome for consecutive two menstrual cycle (2) Severe depression or no depression as measured by the IPAT depression scale were excluded from the study. After this preliminary assessment, with the help of a simple random sampling method 1st and 2nd year bachelor degree girls who had fulfilled the inclusion criteria were selected from each college.

3.3 RESEARCH VARIABLES:

Baseline variables:

Demographic variables.

Personal and menstrual variables.

Obstetrical and gynecological variables.

Independent variables:

Foot reflexology technique and Hot foot bath therapy.

Dependent variable:

Premenstrual syndrome and depression.

3.4 SETTING OF THE STUDY

The study was conducted in selected arts and science colleges at Pathanamthitta district, Kerala. The researcher approached the principals of 14 arts and science colleges of Pathanamthitta district to conduct the research study. Nine colleges were agreed to participate in the study. Out of these 9 colleges 6 colleges were selected randomly for either the experimental groups or the control group. The multi-colleges study maximized the chances of obtaining a representative sample of adolescent girls in Pathanamthitta district. The participants received the assigned intervention in the hostel of each of the colleges involved in the study. The outcome measure follow- up was completed at college.

3.5 POPULATION

The target population for the study included the adolescent girls in the age group of 17 to 19 years and studying 1st and 2nd year bachelor degree courses. The accessible population for the study included the adolescent girls who had been having mild, moderate or strong premenstrual syndrome and mild or moderate depression and studying in 1st and 2nd year bachelor degree courses at selected arts and science colleges in Pathanamthitta district.

3.6 SAMPLE

The sample consisted of adolescent girls with premenstrual syndrome and depression and those who fulfilled the inclusion criteria during the period of study at selected arts and science colleges in Pathanamthitta district, and were willing to take part in the study.

3.7 SAMPLE SIZE CALCULATION

Sample size was calculated using the following formula

Equation 3.7.1

$$N = \frac{[(Z\alpha/_2+Z\beta)^2 + (P_1(1-P_1) + P_2(1-P_2))]}{(P_1-}$$

Where

$Z\alpha/_2$ = Z value for $\alpha/_2$ level

$Z\beta$ = Z value β is the power

P_1 = Proportional cure rate in the first group

$1-P_1$ = Number of individuals who did not receive cure in first group

P_2 = Proportional cure rate in the second group

$1-P_2$ = Number of individuals who did not receive cure in second group

$Z\alpha/_2$ is a constant Z value for $\alpha/_2$ level

α error	**5%**	**1%**	**0.1%**
2 Sided	**1.96**	**2.57**	**3.29**
1Sided	**1.65**	**2.33**	

$Z\beta$ is a constant set by convention according to power of the study as below

Power	**80%**	**85%**	**90%**	**95%**
Value	**0.842**	**1.037**	**1.282**	**1.645**

Two proportions are used in situations in which there are two treatments to be compared and we need to know the cure rate in each group

P_1 is the proportion of individual receiving cure rate in group I

P_2 is the proportion of individual receiving cure rate in group II

We need the following values:

$Z\alpha/_2$, $Z\beta$, P1, P2

Let us assume we will accept a $P<0.05$ as acceptable and a study with 80% power.Using the above table we get the following values:

$Z\alpha$ =1.96 (In this case we will be using a two tailed test because the result could be bidirectional).

$Z\beta$ =0.842 (Value of 80% power)

P_1=18% (Proportion of cure rate in foot reflexology)

$1-P_1$=82 % (Proportion of individuals who didn't get cure in foot reflexology)

P_2=22 % (Proportion of cure rate in hot foot bath)

$1-P_2$=78 % (Proportion of individuals who did not get cure in hot foot bath)

The difference of cure rate of two different interventions is 4%

$$N = \frac{[(1.96+0.842)^2 + 0.18(1-0.18) + .22(1-0.22)]}{(0.4)^2}$$

$$N = \frac{7.8512+0.1476+0.1716}{0.16}$$

= 51 subjects /group

A total of 51 subjects/ group were needed to achieve a significance of 0.05 and a power of 0.8 for 18% reduction in foot reflexology and 22% reduction in hot foot bath therapy in the total PMS score. To get a comfortable sample size, considering the possibility of attrition, the researcher decided to enrol 10% excess sample for the study. Hence the sample constituted of 56 subjects per arm. Rounding up to the nearest whole number, the estimated sample size was 60 in each group. Total number of samples for the study was 180.

3.8 SAMPLE SELECTION CRITERIA

3.8.1 Inclusion criteria

Adolescent girls who:

- ❖ were in the age group of 17-19 years
- ❖ had mild, moderate, or strong premenstrual syndrome as measured by the Moos Menstrual Distress Questionnaire (MDQ)
- ❖ had mild or moderate depression as measured by the IPAT questionnaire for depression
- ❖ had been having regular menstrual cycles (28-35 days)
- ❖ were willing to participate in the study
- ❖ no pain medication taken in the previous month before receiving the intervention
- ❖ being able to listen, speak, read, and write English and Malayalam
- ❖ consent for participation received from parent of potential participant under 19 years and potential participant‘s consent to participate in the study

3.8.2 Exclusion Criteria

Adolescent girls who:

- ❖ were unable to participate in the study due to health deviations
- ❖ were physically challenged
- ❖ had severe premenstrual syndrome and severe depression
- ❖ were not having premenstrual syndrome symptoms and depression
- ❖ were having systemic disease such as hypertension, heart disease, diabetes mellitus, renal failure, thrombolytic disease, etc.
- ❖ has any lower extremities infection, injury, disease or open wounds

❖has any prior experience of receiving foot reflexology or hot foot bath therapy

3.9 SAMPLING TECHNIQUE

Fourteen arts and science colleges in Pathanamthitta district were approached and nine colleges were agreed to participate in the study. Out of these 9 colleges 6 colleges were selected using simple random sampling (Lottery method).Then adolescent girls having mild, moderate and strongpremenstrual syndrome with mild or moderate depression were selected using simple random sampling technique.

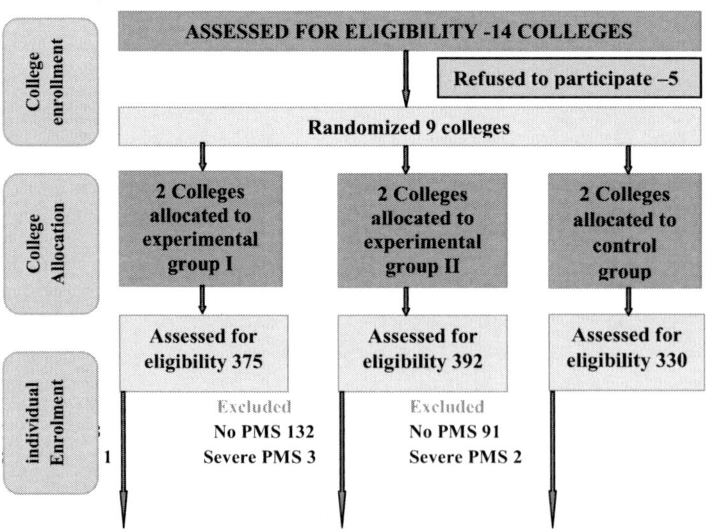

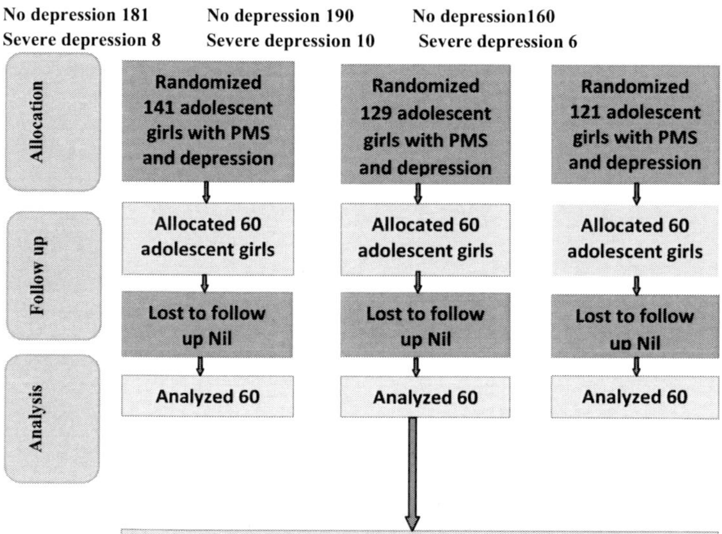

Figure 3.9.1: Flow chart of participant's recruitment

3.10 DEVELOPMENT AND DESCRIPTION OF THE TOOL

Extensive review of literature, discussion and views of experts enhanced the development of the tool; the tool consists of 4 parts.

3.10.1 Part I: Background variable tool

A background variable tool was developed by the researcher to collect data on demographic variables, personal data and gynaecological related study variables. It consists of three sections

Section A: Demographic variables

Demographic variables includes details such as age, class which they study, type of accommodation, educational status of father, educational status of mother, occupation of the father, occupation of the mother, and monthly income of the family.

Section B: Personal data

Personal data of the adolescent girls include; height, weight, BMI, class performance, class attendance, exam missing, and remedial measures taken during menstruation.

Section C: Gynaecological related study variables

Gynaecological related study variables include age at menarche, menstrual regularity, menstrual duration, menstrual interval, menstrual flow, premenstrual syndrome awareness.

Scoring and Interpretation

No score was allotted. The data were used for descriptive analysis. The body mass index was calculated using formula: BMI = weight in kg /height in meter square and classified according to World Healh Organization (WHO).

Administration

The back ground variable questions were answered by adolescent girls during survey andpost-test. The class performance and class attendance were collected from the class coordinators.

3.10.2 Part II: Moos Menstrual Distress Questionnaire (MMDQ)

This standardized form was constructed by Rudolf. H. Moos (1969).The MDQ was used to analyse the behavioural and affective responses of adolescent girls, the items of MDQ were associated with premenstrual, menstrual and post menstrual phases. The questionnaire contains description of symptoms classified in to eight categories (total 47 items) such as pain (6), impaired concentration (9), behavioural change (5), autonomic reaction (4), water retention (4), negative effect (8), arousal (5), and control (6), each of which was scored relating to three different phases of a menstrual cycle. Thus the questionnaire provided score based on 47 variables related to premenstrual syndrome (PMS). The MDQ form c comprised of three separate self-reporting columns to measure common symptoms and feelings associated with premenstrual, menstrual and post menstrual phases. It allows participants to describe their experience and rate the intensity of their experience as follows

0 No experience of symptom 1 Present, mild

2 Present, moderate 3 Present, strong

4 Present, severe

Scoring and Interpretation

Each item had five options categorized on a 0-4 rating scale with scores as mentioned above. The total score was 188. The level of premenstrual syndrome was ranged as follows:

Score	Level of premenstrual syndrome
0	No PMS symptoms
1-47	Mild PMS
48-94	Moderate PMS
95-144	Strong PMS
145-188	Severe PMS

Administration

The MDQ was answered by adolescent girls during survey and post-test. Subjects were asked to report the presence or absence of these symptoms, based on their previous month's menstrual cycle experiences as well as with the help of daily symptom dairy.

3.10.3 Part III–Institute for Personality and Ability Testing (IPAT)Questionnaire for depression

The IPAT depression scale is also known as personal assessment inventory, was created by Samuel Krug and James Laughlin contains 40 statements about how people feel or think at one time or other. Each item is rated with a set of three possible answers. In order to obtain a maximally valid and reliable estimate of depression scale the investigator used the uncorrected scores obtained from 36 items. Scoring is done by using a scoring key sheet for the IPAT depression scale. Place the key over the answer boxes on page 2 and 3 of the booklet centre, the star at the top of the page in the hole so marked and the right edge of the key on the vertical line at the right side of the page. Since the investigator is using uncorrected factor of scoring add 1's and 2's down the page for those items falling within the unshaded portion of the key in the page number two and three and write the total score. This obtained score is the uncorrected raw score. Then convert the raw score into standard score on a 10 point scale. Since this study has conducted among the college students, for converting raw score to standard score the investigator has used the norms for converting raw scores to standard scores for specific groups i.e. college students.

Scoring and Interpretation

The total raw score was 72. The level of depression was grouped as follows:

Raw score	Standard score	Level of depression
0-6	1-3	Mild depression
7-33	4-7	Moderate depression
34-72	8-10	Severe depression

Adolescent girl's scores ranging from 0-6 raw score or 1-3 standard score is mild depression and 7-33 raw score or 4-7 standard score is moderate depression, only were considered for the study.

Administration

The IPAT depression scale questions were answered by adolescent girls during the survey and post-test. Subjects were asked to report the presence or absence of these symptoms, based on their past two month's experiences during luteal phase as well as with the help of daily symptom dairy.

3.10.4 Part 1V- Daily symptom dairy

Maintenance of premenstrual daily symptom diary was practised for prospective record of symptoms. This consists of the horizontal columns from the first day to 30th day of the month and vertical columns of 45 symptoms commonly expressed by adolescent girls with PMS. The diary was prepared by the researcher based on the Moos Menstrual Distress Questionnaire.

Adolescent girls were requested to record their symptoms at the end of the day, during evenings as mild, moderate, strong or severe, if no

symptoms were there the space for that day was left blank and they were also instructed to mark the first menstrual day in red pen. The researcher described the daily symptom diary and taught them how to record symptoms in the daily record. Weekly, the researcher reminded the adolescent girls about keeping the daily symptom diary. Adolescent girls maintained daily symptom diary throughout the study period.

Scoring and administration

Students were requested to fill the diary at the end of the day after college hours. As the daily symptom diary was used to identify luteal phase symptoms and also used to complete Moos Menstrual Distress Questionnaire, no scores were assigned to them.

3.11 VALIDITY AND RELIABILITY OF THE TOOL

All the instruments were reviewed for face and content validity by medical and nursing experts and they were pilot tested to assess the usability and ease of administration. Content validity of the tool was established by experts comprising of two educationalists, one psychologist, one psychiatrist, four nurse educators, one reflexology practitioner, and one gynaecologist.

3.11.1 Menstrual distress questionnaire Form c (MDQ)

It is a standardized tool. Re-test reliability of the whole test as well as the eight sub components have been reported. These values range from

r = 0.993 to r = 0.998. The original tool has established validity. The adapted tool was translated into the local language Malayalam and checked by two experienced bilingual researchers. Second, the Malayalam version was back-translated into English to ensure the stability of the meaning of each test item

(Chatterjee, 2006). The Malayalam version of MDQ was tested using the test-retest method at two weeks with a sample of 100 students. The `r' value obtained was 0.96 (significant correlation). Questionnaire was utilized with permission of Psycho press, (purchased).

3.11.2 IPAT Questionnaire for Depression

It is a standardized tool. The original tool has established validity. The adapted tool was translated in to Malayalam and back translated into English. The Malayalam version of IPAT was tested using the test-retest reliability method with a sample of 100 students. The reliability coefficients were obtained with Pearson's product moment correlations, indicating significant correlation (r=0.96).

3.12FOOT REFLEXOLOGY TECHNIQUE

Adolescent girls in experimental group I was grouped in to small groups of 10 and was asked to assemble in the room to perform foot reflexology technique. Foot reflexology was given for experimental group I about 15 minutes once a week for 3 months. A total of 6 groups with 10 adolescent girls in each group were grouped for foot reflexology session. The researcher was performing foot reflexology to each individual.

For the reflexology session, thumb and index fingers were used to work on the feet. Make sure the hands are clean and finger nails must be properly trimmed. Make the person in a comfortable position by lying flat on the bed. First mild massage was given on all feet in a firm and gentle manner. By holding the spine area of the foot, slowly and gently twist/ wring the hands away from each other. Hold the heel of the foot with one hand and the ball of the foot with other hand,rotate the foot clockwise and anticlockwise for few

seconds, make stretching movements, move the toes one by one down towards the heel, and rotate each toe clockwise and anticlockwise for few seconds.These measures loosen up the feet. Then do thumb walking by massaging the thumbs repeatedly from the heel area up through the arch of the foot to the ball of the foot which provides relaxation to the person. Then apply pressure on concerned and specified regions.

Figure 3.12.1

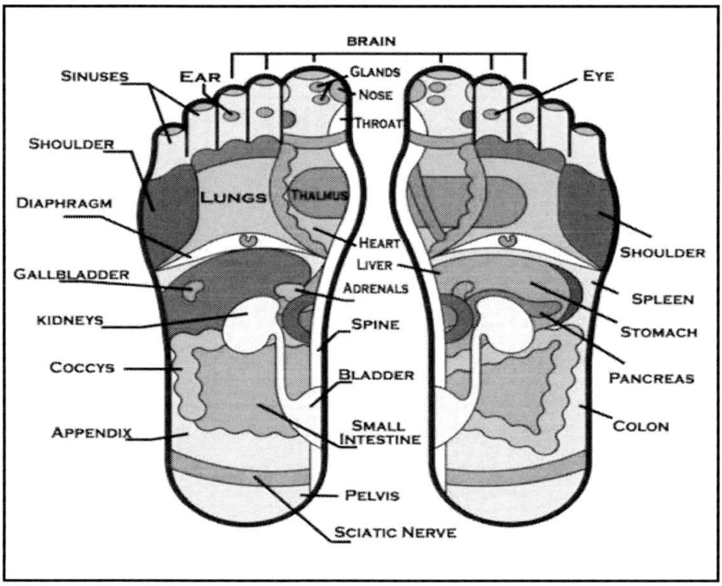

As figure 3.12.1shows, these areas are

Body parts and organs	Corresponding zones at the feet
Spine –very middle of the human body	The most middle aspect of your feet.
Liver - located on the right side of the chest and abdomen	Lateral aspect of right foot

Body parts and organs	Corresponding zones at the feet
Spleen - left side of the ribs, below the heart	Outside or lateral aspect of the left foot.
Head	Located on toes along with all sensory organs
The lower back, sacrum, urinary bladder, genitals and lower limbs	Located towards the heel
Genital zone (ovary and uterus)	Genital zone which include ovarian reflex point and uterine reflex point which located at both feet under the lateral and medial malleolus respectively
Kidneys	Very center of the sole of the foot. depression between the 2nd and 3rd metatarsals, just posterior to the first phalangeal joint

The techniques used for foot reflexology were

Feet preparation: feet were washed with small soft brush for a few minutes. Smoothen the foot with alternating hands forming 3 rounds. Pressed thumbs side-by-side on the heel while other fingers are on the dorsal. Pressedandpulled thumbs straight in the centre of the foot in an upward direction.

Head spin- hands placedloosely on both the sides of forefoot. Hands moved with medium-firm pressure on both the sides of forefeet alternately for 10 times.

Ankle slide–placed heel of hands below anklebones on each side. Pressed the side of the heel and move the hands back and forth in opposite direction.

Ankle rotation- heel held tightly with lower hand while the other hand holding feet from outside. Rotated the foot inward for 5 times using upper hand then outward for 5times.

Ankle massage-with hands holding the foot down to expose the medial side, used thumb to stroke next to anklebone in circular motion for 10 rounds.

Side twist-with both the hands grasp median side of foot, with thumbs pressed on plantar surface of foot. Pressed all fingers while twisting hands back and front in opposite directions alternatively for 5 times.

Foot twist-with one hand holding at heel lower position firmly, used the hand to grasps medial side of upper part foot from outside. With the upper hand twist the foot outwards and change location to cover the entire median side of the foot completing for 5 rounds.

Plantar press-with knuckle facing downpulled downwards from below the ball part of the big toe for 5 rounds. Reverse knuckle face up and pulled upwards to below ball part of the big toe for 5 rounds. Placed thumb near median side to give support. Pulling the knuckle across the ball part towards the big toe for 5 rounds.

Sole massage - pressed thumb side-by-side on the heel while other fingers are on the dorsal. Pressed and pulled thumbs straight in the centre of the foot in an upward direction for 5 times.

Sole press -with thumbs resting on top of each other on the plantar and fingers on the dorsal. Pressed each thumb alternately and moved upward towards the toes and reverse.

Dorsal press -with one hand supporting the foot, knuckle should be pressed on dorsal. Start from the dorsal ankle crease.

Dorsal groove press- with fingers pressing on dorsal grooves next to big toe and little toe and hold it for 10seconds.

Top of foot crease slide -with both thumbs on dorsal ankle creasing it useother fingers to give support under the foot. Press and slide thumbs alternately

Closing- place hands loosely on the dorsal and the plantar and pull alternately for5 rounds.

After the procedure tell to drink plenty of water for the next 24 hours which allows the blood to get rid of waste from the body

3.13 HOT FOOT BATH THERAPY

Adolescent girls in experimental group II were grouped in to small groups of 10 and were asked to assemble in the room to perform hot foot bath therapy. Hot foot bath therapy was given for about 15 minutes once weekly for 3 months. A total of 6 groups with 10 adolescent girls in each group were grouped for hot foot bath session.

- procedure was explained to the patient
- Room should be warm and free of drafts
- Assembled all the equipment and materials to the patients' side
- Better to do hot foot bath treatment on an empty stomach
- Told the patient to drink a glass of warm water before the therapy begins
- Made the patient to sit on a chair comfortably with a cotton cloth covering from chin to below knee, which absorbs all the sweat
- Blanket is covered over the cotton cloth. It should extend all the way to the floor
- A damp towel wraped on the crown and back of the head. Keep it wet throughout the therapy by sprinkling water on it from time to time.

- A towel is covered around patient's neck to absorb sweat and prevent escape of body heat

- Took hot water with a temperature of 100° F to 115° F (43°C- 46°C) in a bucket high enough to cover the ankles
- Checked the temperature of the water before dipping patient's feet in the hot water
- Instructed and assisted the patient to place feet in tub.
- Added hot water as patient can tolerate it, up to 120° F (49°C)
- Removed the feet each time before adding more hot water. Carry on treatment for 5-30 minutes as needed, keeping a cold compress on the patient's head
- It is generally better to start with a lower temperature and gradually increase the temperature of the water
- Continued the treatment until the body is very hot and sweating
- Took feet out of tub; poured ice water over the feet, dried feet, legs and thighs
- After completing the hot foot therapy performed cold friction (rubbing with a cold wet towel on the whole body or take a sponge bath followed by a normal cool bath
- Told the patient to wear thick, warm socks on the feet and told to take rest in bed for minimum of 30 minutes
- Instructed to drink plenty of water.

3.14PILOT STUDY

Prior to starting the main study, a pilot study was conducted to assess whether the foot reflexology and hot foot bath protocols were realistic

and workable, to identify potential practical problems and to identify adverse effects caused by the procedures. The first stage of the pilot study was to assess content validity of the foot reflexology and hot foot bath protocols. The content validity of the intervention protocols were assessed and evaluated by a panel of experts in the area includes two educationalists, one psychologist, one psychiatrist, four nurse educators, one reflexology practitioner, and one gynaecologist.The panel members were asked to evaluate whether individual steps were relevant and appropriate in terms of the specific intervention and to evaluate whether the sequences were suitable for the aim of this study. In addition, the panel members were asked to revise any item that they disagreed with and to identify areas that were not suitably presented. The penal of experts stated that the sequences and steps of foot reflexology and hot foot bath protocol were appropriate, suitable and relevant for the aim of this study.

Following content validity of the intervention protocols, administrative approval was obtained from the principals of arts and science colleges. Three colleges were selected randomly for conducting pilot study and checked prevalence of the PMS among all adolescent girls studying in 1st and 2nd year bachelor degree classes. The researcher used the simple random sampling technique to recruit 60 participants (20 each in experimental group I, II and control), who were fulfilling the sample inclusion criteria. First, the researcher provided information both orally and in writing about the nature of the study to the adolescent girls who stated that they had premenstrual syndrome. Second, immediately after obtaining written consent or assent from participants and consent from their parents the participants were asked to complete the questionnaire including the demographic information questionnaire, MOOS menstrual distress questionnaire and IPAT questionnaire for depression for collecting retrospective symptoms.

Adolescent girls were requested to maintain premenstrual daily symptoms diary from 4th day to 40th day for prospective record of symptoms.The foot reflexology group of 20 adolescent girls from experimental group I was further divided in to 2 groups of 10 students each. The hot foot bath groups of 20 adolescent girls from experimental group II were also further divided in to 2 groups of 10 students each. Both interventions were for 15 minutes once weekly for 3 months to identify any adverse effects, discomforts or concerns regarding the intervention.

The pilot study went very well. All participants were generally comfortable answering all questions. There were no negative written or oral comments about the questionnaire. Participants stated that the instructions and items in the questionnaire were clear. All participants answered the whole questionnaire in an average time of 20-25 minutes. Tools were found to be relevant and feasible to use. There was no confusion, duplication or ambiguity in any questions or tools. Overall study was found to be feasible and no problems were faced. In addition, the participants in both the foot reflexology and hot foot bath group enjoyed the therapy. Though the pilot study demonstrated feasibility some modification were done in the tool as suggested by the experts.

Modifications done after pilot study

Religion was removed from demographic variables as per the ethical and research committee

3.15ETHICAL CONSIDERATION

An approval was obtained from the principals of arts and science colleges in Pathanamthitta district in order to conduct study at their institutions, and also obtained approval from Muthoot Medical Centre College of Nursing ethics committee to conduct the study. The researcher explained about the research activities and procedures, usefulness of the study, confidentiality and privacy assurance and also regarding the permission to withdraw from the study at any time during the study time. The ethical consideration criteria were based on the Indian Council of Medical Research (ICMR) guidelines on biomedical research in human beings. Information essential for consent included description of the purpose of the study, the research activities and the usefulness of the study outcome, assurance of anonymity, privacy and confidentiality, the opportunity to answer any questions that a potential subject might have and the option to withdraw from the study at any time.

3.16DATA COLLECTION PROCEDURE

After obtaining permission from the head of the institutions and after explaining the purpose of the study, written informed consent from the participants, were collected. The data collection procedure was conducted from September 2016 to July 2018

The data were collected in two phases:

First phase data collection was done for experimental groups in two settings

Survey phase

1. After assigning colleges to either experimental groups or control group, a complete survey was done among 1st and 2nd year bachelor degree girls to identify adolescent girls who fulfilled the inclusion criteria. On the first day a detailed summary of the proposed study was informed to the adolescent girls and consent form was given to read. Students were given the opportunity to ask any further questions and then made to sign the consent form. As students were minors aged between 17-19 years, they were requested to get consent from the parents too. On the third day consent forms were collected from the students and then MDQ and IPAT depression questionnaire were handed over and requested to recall their previous month premenstrual phase experience retrospectively to fill the form and after 20 minutes forms were collected back. This retrospective assessment was done to assess premenstrual syndrome and depression.

2. After the first retrospective assessment, adolescent girls were requested to maintain premenstrual daily symptoms diary from 4th day to 40th day for prospective record of symptoms, the researcher described the daily symptom diary and taught them how to record the symptom in the daily record. Adolescent girls were instructed to record the symptoms for one menstrual cycle in the evening. Weekly the researcher reminded the adolescent girls about keeping the daily symptom diary. 40 days after the first visit, the same adolescent girls were asked to complete a baseline assessment using the completed daily symptom diary. Thus, the baseline assessment included the data from two consecutive menstrual cycles (Diagnosis of PMS need symptom assessment from two consecutive menstrual cycles).

3. These retrospective and prospective cross sectional data were used to identity adolescent girls with mild, moderate, or strong premenstrual syndrome and mild or moderate depression. Based on this preliminary assessment, the adolescent girls excluded from the study were those who had (1) severe premenstrual syndrome as measured by Moos Menstrual Distress Questionnaire or no premenstrual syndrome for consecutive two menstrual cycles (2) severe depression or no depression as measured by the IPAT questionnaire for depression. After this preliminary assessment, a list was prepared comprising 1st and 2nd year bachelor degree girls. With the help of simple random sampling method, 30 adolescent girls were selected from each college.

In the first college among the experimental group I, out of 200 adolescent girls surveyed a total of 116 adolescent girls had premenstrual syndrome and depressive symptoms, in 2nd college out of 175 adolescent girls surveyed a total of 91 adolescent girls had premenstrual syndrome and depressive symptoms. Among the colleges of the experimental group II, in the first college 200 students were surveyed and a total of 109 adolescent girls had premenstrual syndrome and depressive symptoms. In the 2nd college out of 192 adolescent girls surveyed a total of 87 adolescent girls had premenstrual syndrome and depressive symptoms. The colleges which had selected as control group,in the first college 178 adolescent girls surveyed and 91 girls had premenstrual syndrome with depression and in the second college 152 girls surveyed and 86 girls got premenstrual syndrome with depression. After this preliminary assessment a list was prepared separately of each college and by using simple random method, 30 adolescent girls were selected from each college for the study.

Data collection phase

4. After selecting 30 students each from 6 colleges who were fulfilling the inclusion criteria, 60 students from 2 colleges were selected as experimental group I,60 students from next 2 colleges were selected as samples of experimental group II and 60 students from remaining 2 colleges were selected as control group samples. Colleges were selected randomly to different groups. Survey score itself used as pretest score for depression and premenstrual syndrome.

Intervention phase for the adolescent girls

5. After the pretest, samples from experimental group I undergone foot reflexology for 15 minutes once a week for 3 months and experimental group II samples were undergone hot foot bath therapy for 15 minutes once a week for 3 months.

6. The intervention group of 60 adolescent girls from experimental group I was further divided in to 6 groups of 10 students each. The foot reflexology techniques were performed by the researcher herself for each sample and it took place weekly six days in the adolescent girls' hostel during evening time after the college hours. The intervention groups of 60 adolescent girls from experimental group II were also further divided in to 6 groups of 10 students each. The hot foot bath therapy was given by the

researcher to these samples and it took place weekly six days in the adolescent girls' hostel in the morning time before the college hours. Both interventions were for 15 minutes once weekly for 3 months. Two weeks after completing the interventions all the groups were asked to complete the post test form for assessing premenstrual syndrome and depression.

The second phase data collection was done for the control group

60 adolescent girls of control groups were asked to continue their routine activities and were requested to complete the assessments at the same time intervals as the experimental groups. The control group subjects were taught the same intervention at the completion of the study period. The details of the control group participants are as follows; the colleges which had selected as control group, in thefirst college178 adolescent girls surveyed and 91 girls had PMS with depression and in the second college 152 girls surveyed and 86 girls got PMS with depression. Using a simple random sampling technique 30 adolescent girls was selected from each college as samples of control group.

There were no drop outs or attrition of samples from any of the three groups.

Table: 3.16.1 SCHEMATIC REPRESENTATION OF DATA COLLECTION PROCEDURE

Visit day details	Activities Survey phase	Group
1^{st}day	Informed consent from adolescent girls and their parents were handed over to all adolescent girls	Exp. I, II & Control group
3rd day	Adolescent girls were requested to fill background variable form, MDQ form and	Exp.I, II & Control

	IPAT depression questionnaire to collect preliminary retrospective data to assess level of premenstrual syndrome and depression of previous menstrual cycle.	group

Table: 3.16.1 Contd/

Visit day details	Activities Survey phase	Group
4th to 40th day (weekly once)	Reminder to maintain PMS daily symptom dairy every day in the evening to record the symptoms prospectively	Exp.I, II & Control group
41st day	Adolescent girls requested to fill MDQ and IPAT form for depression with the help of daily symptom dairy to record prospective data for one menstrual cycle (diagnosis of PMS need data from 2 cycles). After preliminary assessment a list of adolescent girls who had fulfilled the inclusion criteria were prepared and using a simple random sampling technique, needed numbers of adolescent girls were selected for the study.	Exp. group I, II & Control group
1st day	**Data collection phase** Pre-test score for premenstrual syndrome and depression were taken from the prospective survey score itself	Exp. I, II & Control group
2nd day to 90th day	Performing foot reflexology technique for study group I (once weekly 15 minutes for 3 months)	Exp. group I
	Giving hot foot bath therapy for study group	Exp. group II

	II(once weekly 15 minutes for 3 months)	
	Routine measures	Control group
2 weeks after the intervention	Post test assessment of premenstrual syndrome and depression	Exp. I, II & Control group

3.17 DATA ANALYSIS PLAN

Descriptive statistics was used to arrange the data in a scientific way. Inferential statistics was used to test the hypothesis. Data were analysed using the Statistical Package for the Social Sciences (SPSS version 20). A p value of < 0.05 was considered significant

Table 3.17.1 Plan for data analysis

Methods	Type of statistics	Purpose
Descriptive statistics	Frequency, Percentage, Mean, SD	Assess the sample characteristics and study variables.
Inferential Statistics	Paired 't' test	Compare the outcome variables before and after intervention within the group
	Independent 't' test	Compare the outcome variables before and after intervention between the groups.
	Chi square	Assess the homogeneity of samples between the groups. Associate selected background variables with outcome variables.
	ANOVA	Associate selected background variables with outcome

		variables.
	Multiple Linear Regressions	All the significant variables were grouped into final regression analysis to evaluate the role of the different independent variables on the dependent variable.

CHAPTER IV

DATA ANALYSIS AND INTERPRETATION

This chapter deals with the analysis and interpretation of data collected in selected arts and science colleges of Pathanamthitta district to compare the effectiveness of foot reflexology and hot foot bath therapy on premenstrual syndrome and depression among adolescent girls. The responses were tabulated and analysed under the following sections according to the sequence of the study objectives stated.

Section- 4.1: Prevalence of premenstrual syndrome and depression among adolescent girls at six selected arts and science colleges in Pathanamthitta district (Tables: 4.1.1 to 4.1.2 and figures 4.1.1to 4.1.2)

Section- 4.2: Distribution of study related background variables among adolescent girls in the experimental group I, II and control group (Tables: 4.2.1 to 4.2.3 and figures 4.2.1.1 to 4.2.1.8, 4.2.2.1 to 4.2.2.5, and 4.2.3.1 to 4.2.3.6)

Section- 4.3: Comparison of premenstrual syndrome and depression within the groups and between the groups (Tables: 4.3.1to 4.3.29 and figures 4.3.1to 4.3.8)

Section- 4.4: Association of selected background variables with outcome variables of adolescent girls in the experimental group I, II and control group (Tables: 4.4.1 to 4.4.6)

Section-4.5: Regression of selected outcome variables with selected background variables among adolescent girls in the experimental group I, II and control group (Tables: 4.5.1 to 4.5.6)

Section-4.1: Prevalence of PMS and depression among adolescent girls at six selected arts and science colleges in Pathanamthitta district

Table 4.1.1: Prevalence (%) of premenstrual syndrome (PMS) among adolescent girls at six selected arts and science colleges in Pathanamthitta district (n=1097)

Premenstrual syndrome	No	%
No PMS	331	30.17
Mild	399	36.37
Moderate	335	30.54
Strong	26	2.37
Severe	6	0.55

Table 4.1.1 shows that 331 (30.17%) adolescent girls did not have premenstrual syndrome. 399 (36.37%) had mild premenstrual syndrome and 335 (30.54%) adolescent girls had moderate level of premenstrual syndrome. Strong premenstrual syndrome was found among 26 (2.37%) adolescent girls. 6 (0.55%) adolescent girls had severe premenstrual syndrome.

Table 4.1.2: Prevalence (%) of depression among adolescent girls at six selected arts and science colleges in Pathanamthitta district (n=1097)

Premenstrual depression	No	%
No Depression	531	48.41
Mild	132	12.03
Moderate	410	37.37
Severe	24	2.19

Table 4.1.2 depicts that 531 (48.41%) adolescent girls did not have premenstrual depression. 132 (12.03%) and 410 (37.37%) adolescent girls had

mild and moderate level of premenstrual depression respectively. Severe premenstrual depression was found among 24 (2.19%) adolescent girls.

Figure 4.1.1: Prevalence (%) of premenstrual syndrome among adolescent girls at six selected arts and science colleges in Pathanamthitta district (n=1097)

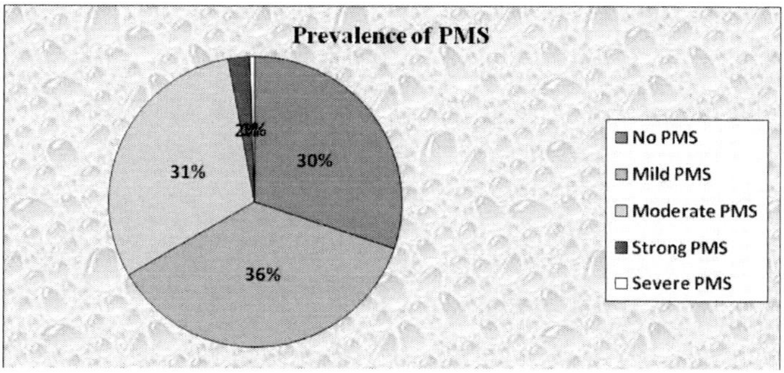

Figure 4.1.2: Prevalence (%) of depression among adolescent girls at six selected arts and science colleges in Pathanamthitta district (n=1097)

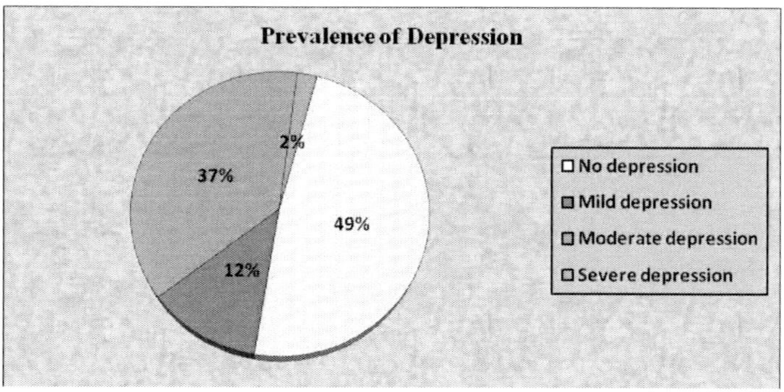

Section-4.2: Distribution of study related background variables among adolescent girls in the experimental group I, II and control group

Table 4.2.1: Frequency, percentage and chi square distribution of demographic variables among adolescent girls in the experimental group I, II and control group (n=180)

Demographic variables	Experimental group I (n-60)		Experimental group II (n-60)		Control group (n-60)		χ^2 p value
	No	%	No	%	No	%	
Age (in years)							
16-17	11	18.33	12	20	9	15	0.532
18-19	49	81.67	48	80	51	85	0.766NS
Class of studying							
1st Year	33	55	22	36.67	31	51.67	4.587
2nd Year	27	45	38	63.33	29	48.33	1.101 NS
Place of residence							
Hostel	26	43.33	13	21.67	22	36.67	6.596
Home	34	56.67	47	78.33	38	63.33	.037*S
Educational status of father							
Primary	5	8.33	1	1.67	2	3.33	12.329
High school	14	23.33	26	43.33	20	33.33	0.137NS
H. Secondary	19	31.67	12	20	18	30	
Graduate	16	26.67	17	28.33	19	31.67	
Post graduate	6	10	4	6.67	1	1.67	
Educational status of mother							
Primary	3	5	1	1.67	3	5	5.461
High school	15	25	23	38.33	22	36.66	0.707 NS
H.Secondary	20	33.33	16	26.67	16	26.67	
Graduate	18	30	17	28.33	16	26.67	
Post graduate	4	6.67	3	5	3	5	

Table 4.2.1 Contd/-

Demographic variables	Experimental group I (n-60)		Experimental group II (n-60)		Control group (n-60)		χ2 p value
	No	%	No	%	No	%	
Occupation of the father							
Unemployed	3	5	5	8.33	1	1.67	7.829
Unskilled worker	11	18.33	4	6.67	9	15	0.251NS
Skilled worker	10	16.67	16	26.67	11	18.33	
Professional	36	60	35	58.33	39	65	
Occupation of the mother							
Housewife	43	71.67	52	86.67	48	80	4.240
Skilled worker	3	5	1	1.67	2	3.33	0.374 NS
Professional	14	23.33	7	11.66	10	16.67	
Family income (Rs./month)							
<2500 -2500	11	18.33	20	33.33	11	18.33	13.061
2501- 5000	5	8.33	4	6.67	7	11.67	0.109NS
5001-7500	6	10	12	20	5	8.33	
7501-10000	19	31.67	12	20	22	36.67	
10001 ->10001	19	31.67	12	20	15	25	

S Significant, NS Non significant, *p <.05

Descriptive analysis of the demographic variables indicated that 11 (18.33%) in the experimental group I, 12 (20%) in the experimental group II and 9 (15%) in the control group belongs to the age group of 16-17 years. Majority of them, 49 (81.67%) in the experimental group I, 48 (80%) in the experimental group II and 51 (85%) in the control group were in the age group of 18-19 years.

Regarding the class of studying 33 (55%) in the experimental group I, 22 (36.67%) in the experimental group II and 31 (51.67%) in the control group were studying in first year bachelor degree course. 27 (45%) in the

experimentalgroup I, 38 (63.33%) in the experimental group II and 29 (48.33%) in the control group were in the 2nd year bachelor degree classes.

Regarding the educational status of the fathers, 5 (8.33%) in the experimental group I, and 1 (1.67%) in the experimental group II and 2 (3.33%) in the control group had primary education. 14 (23.33%) in the experimental group I, 26 (43.33%) in the experimental group II and 20 (33.33%) in the control group had completed their high school education.19(31.67%) in the experimental group I, 12 (20%) in the experimental group II and 18 (30%) in the control group had completed their higher secondary education.16 (26.67%), 17 (28.33%) and 19 (31.67%) in the experimental group I,experimental group II and the control group were graduates respectively. 6 (10%) in the experimental group I, 4 (6.67%) in the experimental group II and 1 (1.67%) in the control group had completed their post-graduation degree.

With respect to educational status of the mother 3 (5%) in the experimental group I, 1 (1.67%) in the experimental group II and 3 (5%) in the control group had completed primary education. 15 (25%) in the experimental group I, 23 (38.33%) in the experimental group II and 22 (36.66%) in the control group had completed high school education. 20 (33.33%) in the experimental group I, 16 (26.67%) each in experimental group II and control group were completed higher secondary education. 18 (30%) in the experimental group I, 17 (28.33%) in the experimental group II and 16 (26.67%) in the control group were graduates. 4 (6.67%) in the experimental group I, 3 (5%) each in the experimental group II and the control group were post graduates.

113

Regarding the occupation of fathers 3(5%) in the experimental group I, 5 (8.33%) in the experimental group II and 1(1.67%) in control group were unemployed. 11(18.33%) in the experimental group I and 4 (6.67%) in the experimental group II, 9 (15%) in the control group were unskilled workers. 10(16.67%) in the experimental group I ,16 (26.67%) in the experimental group II, and 11 (18.33%) in the control group were skilled workers. Majority of them 36 (60%), 35 (58.33%), 39 (65%) in the experimental group I, II and control group were professionals respectively.Regarding the occupation of mothers majority of them 43(71.67%), 52(86.67%), 48(80%) in the experimental group I, II and control experimental group were house wives respectively. 3 (5%) in the experimental group I,1(1.67%) in the experimental group II and 2 (3.33%)in the control group were skilled workers.14(23.33%) in the experimental group I,7(11.67%) in the experimental group II and 10 (16.67%) in the control group were professionals.

The total family income per month highlighted that11 (18.33%) each in the experimental group I and control group and 20(33.33%) in the experimental group II had family income range of Rs. <2500-2500. 5 (8.33%) in the experimental group I, 4(6.67%) in the experimental group II and 7 (11.66%) in the control group had a family income range of Rs. 2501 - 5000 per month. This signified that nearly half of the adolescent girls were from lower middle class family. 6 (10%) in the experimental group I, 12 (20%) in the experimental group II and 5 (8.33%) in the control group had a family income range of Rs. 5001-7500. 19 (31.67%) in the experimental group I, 12 (20%) in the experimental group II and 22(36.67%) in the control group had a family income range of Rs. 7501-10000. 19 (31.67%) in the experimental group I and 12 (20%) in the experimental group II and 15 (25%) in the control

group had a family income range of Rs. >10001.The chi square revealed homogeneity between the experimental group I, II and the control group with regard to all the demographic variables except for place of residence where a dispersion at $p < 0.05$ was noted between the groups.

Figure 4.2.1.1: Percentage distribution of age among adolescent girls in the experimental group I, II and control group

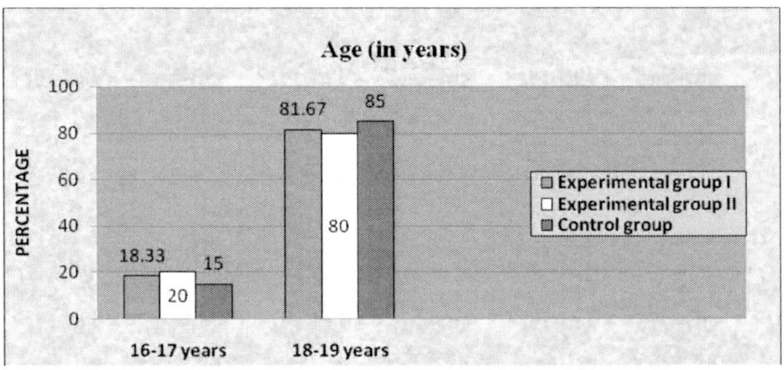

Figure 4.2.1.2: Percentage distribution of class of studying among adolescent girls in the experimental group I, II and control group

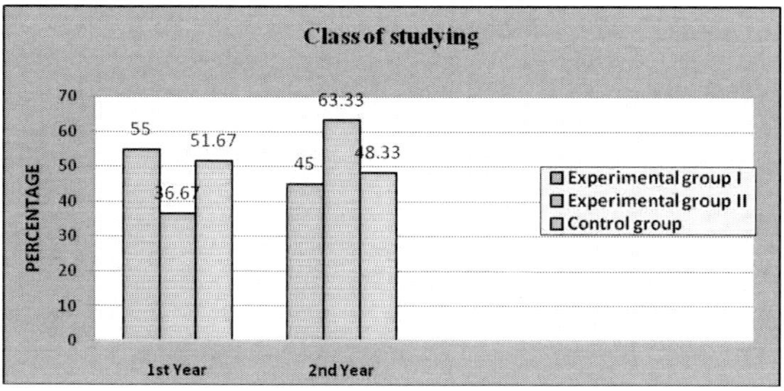

Figure 4.2.1.3: Percentage distribution of place of residence among adolescent girls in the experimental group I, II and control group

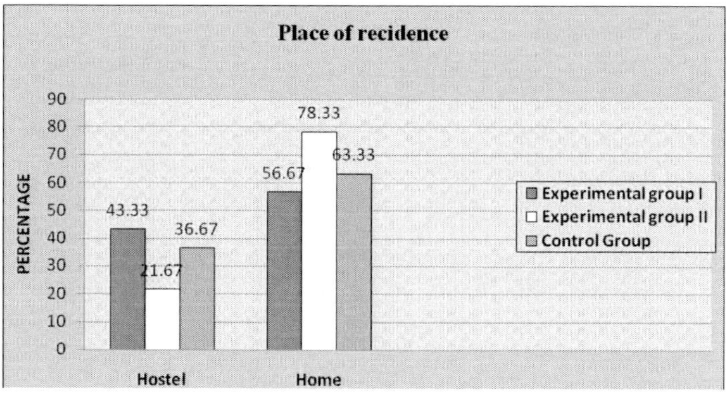

Figure 4.2.1.4: Percentage distribution of education of father among adolescent girls in the experimental group I, II and control group

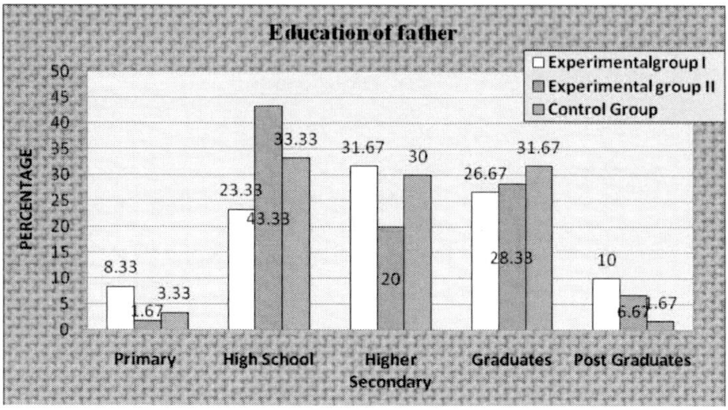

Figure 4.2.1.5: Percentage distribution of education of mother among adolescent girls in the experimental group I, II and control group

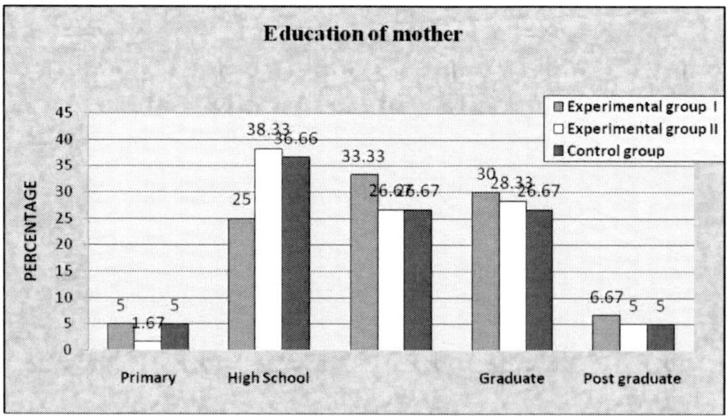

Figure 4.2.1.6: Percentage distribution of occupation of father among adolescent girls in the experimental group I, II and control group

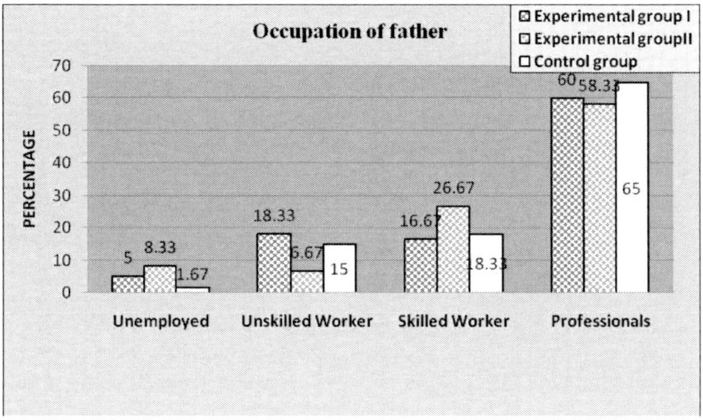

Figure 4.2.1.7: Percentage distribution of occupation of mother among adolescent girls in the experimental groupI, II and control group

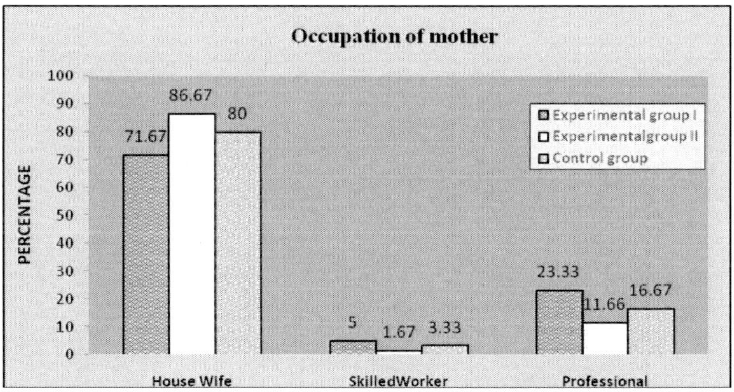

Figure 4.2.1.8: Percentage distribution of monthly income among adolescent girls in the experimental group I, II and control group

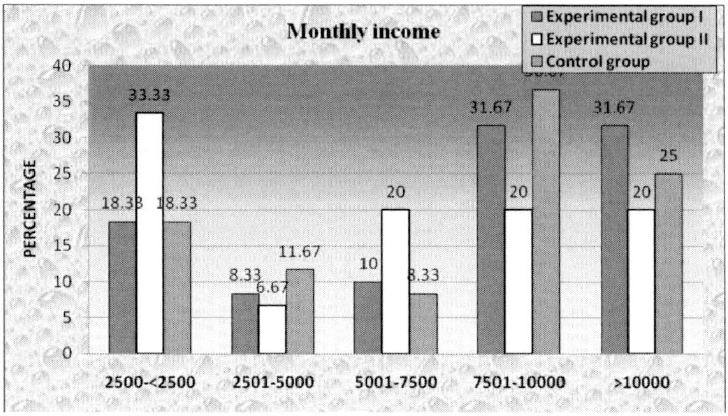

Table 4.2.2: Frequency, percentage and chi square distribution of personal variables among adolescent girls in the experimental group I, II and control group

Personal variables	Experimental group I (n-60)		Experimental group II (n-60)		Control group (n-60)		$\chi 2$ p value
	No	%	No	%	No	%	
BMI							
Under weight	19	31.67	21	35	31	51.67	5.768
Normal	41	68.33	39	65	29	48.33	0.050*S
Class performance							
Good	32	53.33	22	36.67	37	61.67	7.779
Average	28	46.67	38	63.33	23	38.33	0.020*S
Class missing							
Never	28	46.67	34	56.67	34	56.66	1.875
Sometimes	30	50	25	41.67	25	41.67	0.759NS
Always	2	3.33	1	1.67	1	1.67	
Exam missing							
No	11	18.33	6	10	13	21.67	3.12
Yes	49	81.67	54	90	47	78.33	0.210NS

Remedial measures							
Yes	13	21.67	18	30	20	33.33	2.134
No	47	78.33	42	70	40	66.67	0.197NS

S Significant, NS Non Significant, *p<.05

Distribution of personal variables indicated that (Table 4.2.2) nearly half of the adolescent girls 41(68.33%) in the experimental group I, 39(65%) in the experimental group II and 29 (48.33%) in the control group had normal weight. 19(31.67%) in the experimental group I, 21 (35%) in the experimental group II and 31 (51.67%) in the control group had underweight.The class performance of adolescent girls revealed that 32(53.33%) in the

experimental group I, 22(36.67%) in the experimental group II and 37(61.67%) in the control group were having good performance.28 (46.67%)in the experimental group I, 38(63.33%) in the experimental group II and 23 (38.33%) in the control group were having fair performance in the class.

Regarding the class absenteeism 28 (46.67%) in the experimental group I,34 (56.66%) each in the experimental group II and control group respectively had never missed their classes during menstruation. 30(50%) in the experimental group I, 25 (41.66%) in the experimental group II and 25 (41.66%) in the control group had missed their classes during menstruation.
2 (3.33%) in the experimental group I and 1(1.67%) each in the experimental group II and control group were always missing their classes during menstruation.

Exam missing of the adolescent girls during menstruation revealed that 11(18.33%) in the experimental group I, 6(10%) in the experimental group II and 13 (21.67%) in the control group were missing exams during menstruation and remaining girls were not missing their classes during menstruation.13(21.67%) adolescent girls in the experimental group I, 18 (30%) in the experimental group II and 20 (33.33%) in the control group were using some or other remedial measures to control premenstrual syndrome symptoms.

The chi square revealed homogeneity between the groups with regard to all the personal variablesexcept for BMI and class performance where a dispersion at $p < 0.05$ wasnoted between the groups.

Figure 4.2.2.1: Percentage distribution of BMI among adolescent girls in the experimental group I, II and control group

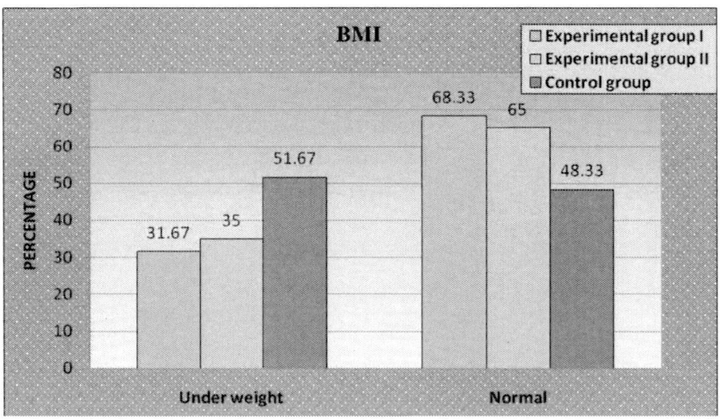

Figure 4.2.2.2: Percentage distribution of class performance among adolescent girls in the experimental group I, II and control group

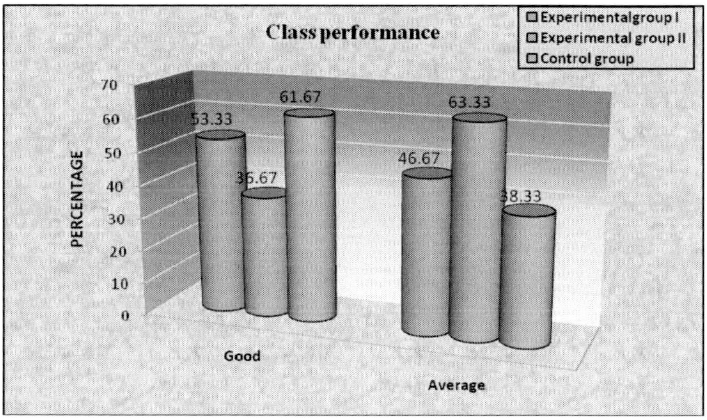

Figure 4.2.2.3: Percentage distribution of class missing among adolescent girls in the experimental group I, II and control group

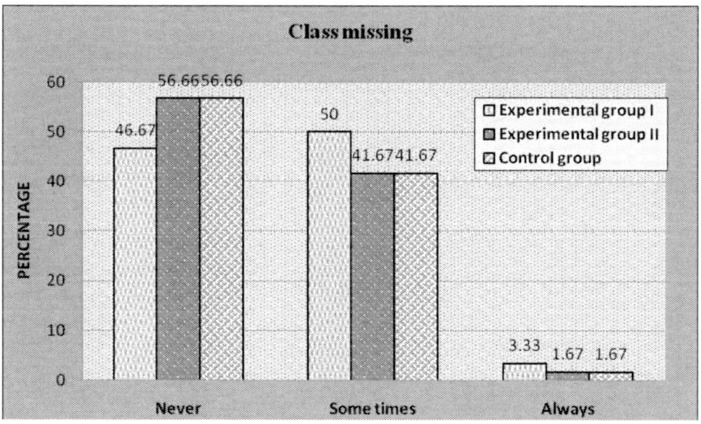

Figure 4.2.2.4: Percentage distribution of exam missing among adolescent girls in the experimental group I, II and control group

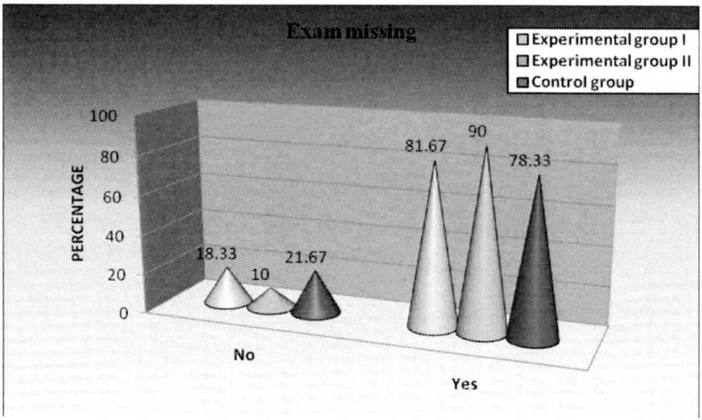

Figure 4.2.2.5: Percentage distribution of remedial measures taken among adolescent girls in the experimental group I, II and control group

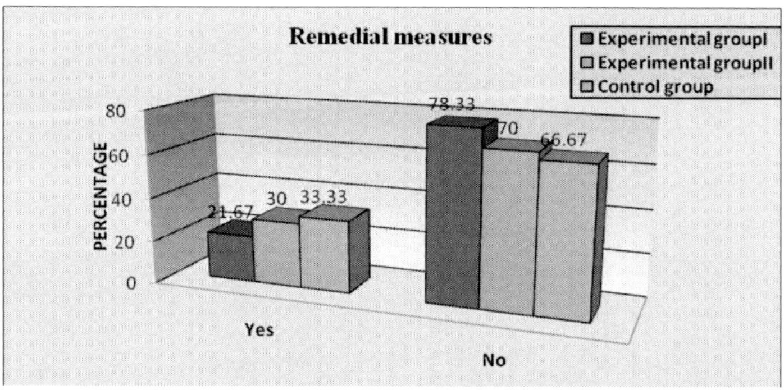

Table 4.2.3: Frequency, percentage and chi square distribution of gynaecological variables among adolescent girls in the experimental group I, II and control group

Gynecological variables	Experimental group I (n-60)	Experimental group II (n-60)	Control group (n-60)	$\chi 2$ p value

	No	%	No	%	No	%	
Ageat menarche							
10-11 years	2	3.33	4	6.67	7	11.67	4.867
12-13 years	37	61.67	31	51.67	35	58.33	0.561NS
14-15 years	20	33.33	23	38.33	17	28.33	
>16 years	1	1.67	2	3.33	1	1.67	
Regularity of menstruation							
Yes	49	81.67	53	88.33	49	81.67	1.315
No	11	18.33	7	11.67	11	18.33	0.518NS
Menstrual duration							
1-2 days	2	3.33	1	1.67	1	1.67	0.819
3-4 days	31	51.67	33	55	30	50	0.936NS
5-6 days	27	45	26	43.33	29	48.33	

Table 4.2.3 Contd/-

Gynecological variables	Experimental group I (n-60)		Experimental group II (n-60)		Control group (n-60)		$\chi 2$ p value
	No	%	No	%	No	%	
Menstrual interval							
15-20 days	3	5	3	5	1	1.67	
21-25 days	19	31.67	12	20	26	43.33	8.502
26-30 days	34	56.66	39	65	28	46.67	0.204NS
31-35 days	4	6.67	6	10	5	8.33	
Menstrual flow							
Light	4	6.67	7	11.67	7	11.67	3.685
Medium	52	86.66	47	78.33	44	73.33	0.450NS
Heavy	4	6.67	6	10	9	15	
PMS awareness							
No	27	45	36	60	28	46.67	3.245
Yes	33	55	24	40	32	53.33	0.197NS

S Significant NS Non Significant

Distribution of gynaecological variables among adolescent girls showed that 2 (3.33%) in the experimental group I and 4 (6.67%) in the experimental group II and 7(11.67%) in the control group attained menarche at the age of 10-11 years. Most of them, 37 (61.67%) adolescent girls in the experimental group I, 31(51.67%) in the experimental group II and 35 (58.33%) in the control group attained menarche at 12-13 years. 20(33.33%) in the experimental group I, 23 (38.34%) in the experimental group II and 17 (28.33%) in the control group adolescents had attained menarche at 14-15years. Remaining attained menarche after 16 years of age.With regard to menstrual duration, 2 (3.33%) girls in the experimental group I and 1(1.67%) each in the experimental group II and control group had menstrual bleeding for 1-2 days. Majority of the girls, 31 (51.67%), 33 (55%), and 30(50%)

adolescent girls had menstrual bleeding for 3-4 days in experimental group I, II and control group respectively. 27(45%) in the experimental group I, 26(43.33%) in the experimental group II and 29(48.33%) in the control group had menstrual bleeding for 5-6 days. Regarding menstrual regularity majority of the adolescent girls 49(81.67%) each in experimental group I and control group and 53(88.33%) in experimental group II had regular menstrual cycle and remaining girls were having irregularity in menstruation.

With regard to menstrual interval 3(5%) adolescent girls in the experimental group I, 3 (5%) in the experimental group II and 1 (1.67%) in the control group had menstrual interval of 15-20 days. 19 (31.67%) in the experimental group I, 12 (20%) in the experimental group II and 26 (43.33%) in control group had menstrual interval of 21-25 days. Most of them 34(56.66%) in experimental group I, 39 (65%) in experimental group II and 28(46.67%) in control group had menstrual interval of 26-30 days.4 (6.67%)

in experimental group I, 6 (10%) in the experimental group II and 5 (8.33%) in the control group had menstrual interval of 31-35 days.

4(6.67%) in experimental group I, 7 (11.67%) each in the experimental group II and control group had light menstrual flow. Most of them, 52(86.66%) in experimental group I, 47 (78.33%) in the experimental group II and 44(73.33%) in control group had medium menstrual flow. 4(6.67%) in experimental group I, 6(10%) in experimental group II and 9 (15%) in control group had heavy menstrual blood flow.PMS awareness highlighted that majority of adolescent girls 27(45%) in experimental group I, 36(60%) in experimental group II and 28(46.67%) in the control group were aware of premenstrual syndrome. The chi square revealed no significant dispersionbetween the groups with regard to the gynaecological variables.

Figure 4.2.3.1: Percentage distribution of age at menarche among adolescent girls in the experimental group I, II and control group

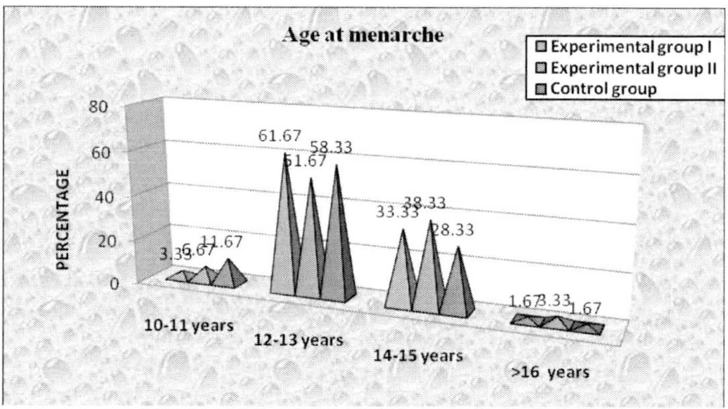

Figure 4.2.3.2: Percentage distribution of menstrual regularity among adolescent girls in the experimental group I, II and control group

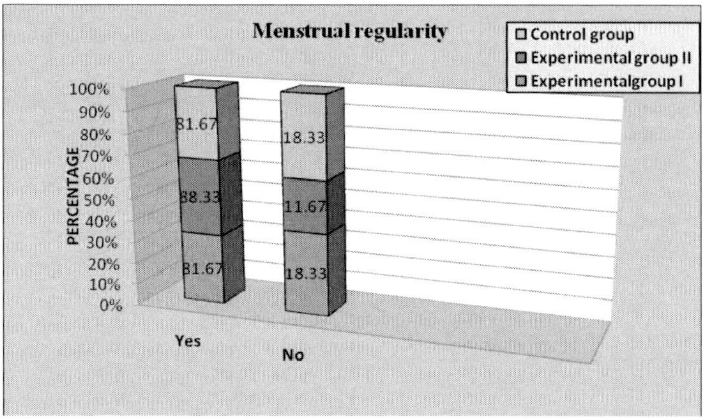

126

Figure 4.2.3.3: Percentage distribution of menstrual interval among adolescent girls in the experimental group I, II and control group

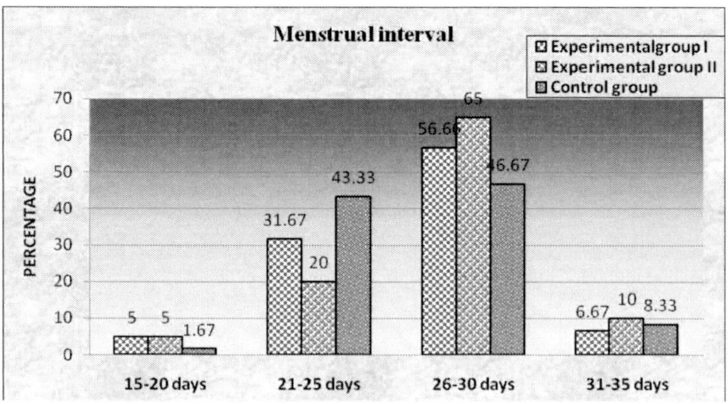

Figure 4.2.3.4: Percentage distribution of menstrual duration among adolescent girls in the experimental group I, II and control group

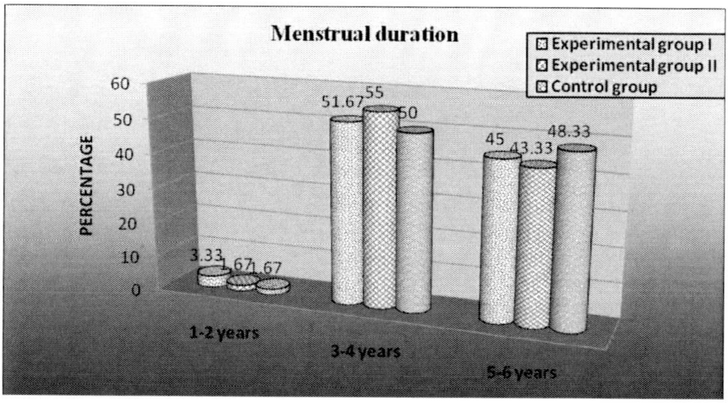

Figure 4.2.3.5: Percentage distribution of menstrual flow among adolescent girls in the experimental group I, II and control group

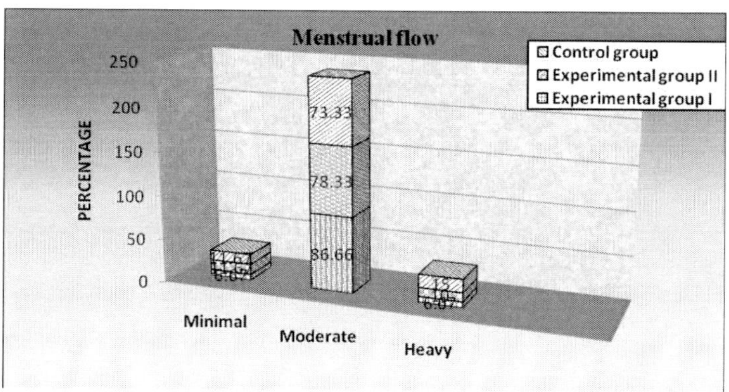

Figure 4.2.3.6: Percentage distribution of PMS awareness among adolescent girls in the experimental group I, II and control group

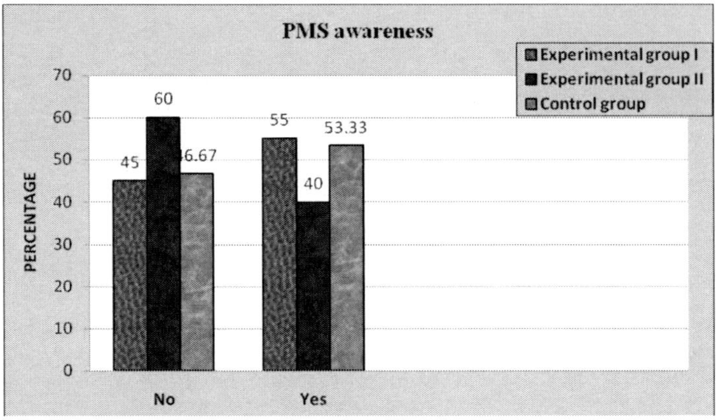

Section-4.3: Comparison of premenstrual syndrome (PMS) and depression within the groups and between the groups

Table 4.3.1: Comparison of level of PMS among adolescent girls in the experimental group I and control group during pre and post-test (n=120)

Level of PMS	Experimental group-I (n=60)		Control group (n=60)		$\chi2$ p value
Pre-test	**No**	**%**	**No**	**%**	
Mild	22	36.67	23	38.34	1.735
Moderate	36	60	35	58.33	0.784NS
Strong	2	3.33	2	3.33	
Post test					
Mild	39	65	20	33.33	12.452
Moderate	19	31.67	38	63.34	.002**S

Strong	2	3.33	2	3.33

S Significant NS Non Significant, ** p <.01

Table 4.3.1 presents the comparison of pre-test premenstrual syndrome level among adolescent girls in the experimental group I and control group. 22 (36.67%) adolescent girls in the experimental group I and 23 (38.33%) adolescent girls in the control group had mild premenstrual syndrome. 36 (60%) adolescent girls in the experimental group I and 35 (58.33%) adolescent girls in the control group had moderate level of premenstrual syndrome. 2 (3.33%) adolescent girls each in the experimental group I and control group had strong premenstrual syndrome. The groups had no significant difference as shown by chi-square value of 1.735 with p value 0.784 between experimental group I and control group. Thus homogeneity between the groups is maintained.

Comparison of post-test premenstrual syndrome level among adolescent girls in the experimental group I and control group reveals that 39 (65%) adolescent girls in the experimental group I and 20 (33.33%) adolescent girls in the control group had mild premenstrual syndrome (PMS). 19 (31.67%) adolescent girls in the experimental group I and 38 (63.34%) adolescent girls in the control group had moderate level of premenstrual syndrome. 2 (3.33%) adolescent girls each in the experimental group I and control group had strong premenstrual syndrome. There is significant difference as shown by chi-square value of 12.452 with p value 0.002 between experimental group I and control group.

Table 4.3.2: Comparison of level of PMS among adolescent girls in the experimental group II and control group during pre-test and post-test (n=120)

Level of PMS	Experimental group II (n=60)		Control group (n=60)		χ2 p value
	No	%	No	%	
Pre test					
Mild	19	31.67	23	38.34	5.450
Moderate	38	63.33	35	58.33	0.244NS
Strong	3	5	2	3.33	
Post test					
Mild	55	91.67	20	3333	17.72
Moderate	5	8.33	38	63.34	0.000***S
Strong	0	0	2	3.33	

S Significant NS Non Significant, ***p<.001

Table 4.3.2 presents the comparison of pre-test premenstrual syndrome level among adolescent girls in the experimental group II and control group.19 (31.67%) girls in the experimental group II and 23 (38.33%)

adolescent girls in the control group had mild premenstrual syndrome (PMS). 38 (63.33%) in experimental group II and 35 (58.33%) adolescent girls in the control group had moderate level of PMS. 3 (5%) adolescent girls in the experimental group II and 2 (3.33%) in the control group had strong PMS. The groups had no significant difference as shown by chi-square value of 5.45 with p value 0.244 between experimental group II and control group. Thus homogeneity between the groups is maintained.

Comparison of post-test premenstrual syndrome level among adolescent girls in the experimental group II and control group reveals that 55 (91.67%) in the experimental group II and 20 (33.33%) adolescent girls in the control group had mild premenstrual syndrome. 5(8.33%) in experimental group II and 38 (63.34%) adolescent girls in the control group had moderate level of PMS. 2 (3.33%) adolescent girls in the control group had strong PMS. There is significant difference as shown by chi square value of 17.72 with p value < 0.001 indicated that there is a significant reduction in the PMS level in the experimental group II than the control group.

Table 4.3.3: Comparison of level of premenstrual syndrome among adolescent girls in the experimental group I and experimental group II during pre-test and post test (n=120)

Level of PMS	**Experimental group I (n=60)**		**Experimental group II (n=60)**		**χ^2 p value**
Pre test	**No**	**%**	**No**	**%**	
Mild PMS	22	36.67	19	38.34	60.614
Moderate	36	60	38	58.33	0.828NS
Strong	2	3.33	3	5	

Table 4.3.3 Contd/.

Level of PMS	**Experimental group I (n=60)**		**Experimental group II (n=60)**		**χ^2 p value**
Post test	**No**	**%**	**No**	**%**	
Mild PMS	39	65	55	91.67	2.197
Moderate	19	31.67	5	8.33	0.032*S
Strong	2	3.33	0	0	

S-Significant, NS Non Significant, *p<.05

Table 4.3.3 presents the comparison of pre-test premenstrual syndrome level among adolescent girls in the experimental group I and experimental group II. 22 (36.67%) adolescent girls in the experimental group

I and 19 (31.67%) in the experimental group II had mild premenstrual syndrome. 36 (60%) adolescent girls in the experimental group I and 38 (63.33%) in experimental group II had moderate level of premenstrual syndrome. 2 (3.33%) adolescent girls in the experimental group I and 3 (5%) adolescent girls in the experimental group II had strong premenstrual syndrome. The groups had no significant difference as shown by chi-square value of 60.614 with p value 0.828 between experimental group I and experimental group II. Thus homogeneity between the groups is maintained.

Comparison of post-test premenstrual syndrome level among adolescent girls in the experimental group I and experimental group II reveals that 39 (65%) adolescent girls in the experimental group I and 55 (91.67%) in the experimental group II had mild premenstrual syndrome (PMS). 19 (31.67%) adolescent girls in the experimental group I and 5 (8.33%) in experimental group II had moderate level of premenstrual syndrome. 2 (3.33%) adolescent girls in the experimental group I had strong premenstrual syndrome. There is significant difference as shown by chi square value of

2.197 with p value <0.05 between experimental group I and experimental group II. A significant statistical difference between the experimental groups indicated that the reduction in the premenstrual syndrome level was better with the experimental group II than the experimental group I.

Table 4.3.4 : Comparison of level of premenstrual syndrome among adolescent girls in the experimental group I, experimental group II and control group during pre-test and post-test (n=180)

Level of PMS	Experimental group-I(n=60)	Experimental group-II(n=60)	Control group (n=60)	$\chi 2$ p value

	No	%	No	%	No	%	
Pre test							
Mild PMS	22	36.67	19	31.67	23	38.34	0.820
Moderate	36	60	38	63.33	35	58.33	0.936NS
Strong	2	3.33	3	5	2	3.33	
Post Test							
Mild PMS	39	65	55	91.67	20	33.3	44.158
Moderate	19	31.67	5	8.33	38	63.34	0.000***S
Strong	2	3.33	0	0	2	3.33	

S-Significant, NS Non Significant, ***p<.001

Table 4.3.4 presents the comparison of pre-test premenstrual syndrome level among adolescent girls in the experimental group I, experimental group II and control group. 22 (36.67%) adolescent girls in the experimental group I, 19 (31.67%) in the experimental group II and 23 (38.34%) in the control group had mild premenstrual syndrome. 36 (60%) adolescent girls in the experimental group I, 38 (63.33%) in experimental group II and 35 (58.33%) in the control group had moderate level of premenstrual syndrome. 2 (3.33%) adolescent girls each in the experimental group I and control group and 3 (5%) adolescent girls in the experimental

group II had strong premenstrual syndromes. The groups had no significant difference as shown by chi-square value of 0.820 with p value 0.936 between experimental group I, experimental group II and control group. Thus homogeneity between the groups is maintained.

Comparison of post-test premenstrual syndrome level among adolescent girls in the experimental group I, experimental group II and control group reveals that 39 (65%) adolescent girls in the experimental group I, 55 (91.67%) in the experimental group II and 20 (33.3%) in the control group had mild premenstrual syndrome. 19 (31.67%) adolescent girls in the experimental group I, 5 (8.33%) in experimental group II and 38 (63.34%) in the control group had moderate level of premenstrual syndrome. 2 (3.33%) adolescent girls each in the experimental group I and control group had strong premenstrual syndrome.

There is significant difference as shown by chi square value of 44.158 with p value <0.001 between experimental group I, experimental group II and control group. A significant statistical difference between the groups indicated that there is a reduction in the PMS level with the experimental group I and II than in the control group.

Figure 4.3.1: Percentage distribution of level of premenstrual syndrome among adolescent girls in the experimental group I during pre-test and post-test.

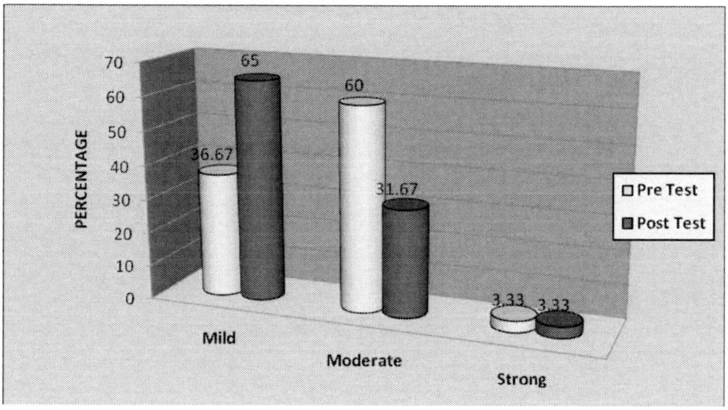

Figure 4.3.2: Percentage distribution of level of premenstrual syndrome among adolescent girls in the experimental group II during pre-test and post- test.

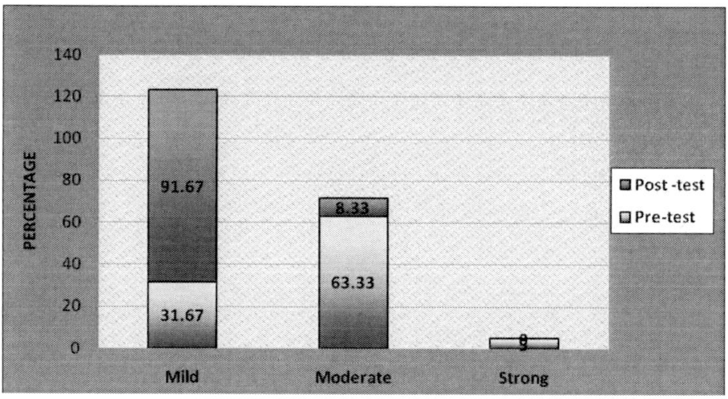

Figure 4.3.3: Percentage distribution of level of premenstrual syndrome among adolescent girls in the control group during pre-test and post- test.

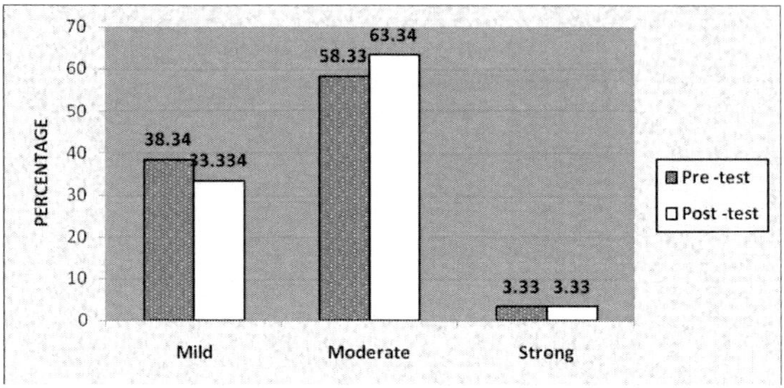

Table 4.3.5 : Comparison of level of depression among adolescent girls in the experimental group I and control group during pre-test and post-test (n=120)

Level of depression	Experimental group-I (n=60)		Control group (n=60)		$\chi 2$ p value
	No	%	No	%	
Pre test					
Mild	8	13.33	8	13.33	0.006
Moderate	52	86.67	52	86.67	0.712NS
Post test					
Mild	9	15	8	13.33	0.424
Moderate	51	85	52	86.67	0.593NS

S-Significant, NS Non Significant

Table 4.3.5 presents the comparison of pre-test depression level among adolescent girls in the experimental group I and control group. 8 (13.33%) adolescent girls each in the experimental group I and control group

had mild depression. Majority of the adolescent girls 52 (86.67%) each in the experimental group I and control group had moderate level of depression. The groups had no significant difference as shown by chi-square value of 0.006 with p value of 0.712 between experimental group I and control group. Thus homogeneity between the groups is maintained.

Comparison of post-test depression level among adolescent girls in the experimental group I and control group reveals that 9 (15%) adolescent girls in the experimental group I and 8 (13.33%) adolescent girls in the control group had mild depression. 51 (85%) adolescent girls in the experimental group I and 52 (86.67%) adolescent girls in the control group had moderate level of depression. There is no significant difference between experimental group I and control group as shown by chi square value of 0.424 with p value 0.593.

Table 4.3.6: Comparison of level of depression among adolescent girls in the exp. group II and control group during pre and post-test (n=120)

Level of depression	Experimental group II (n=60)		Control group (n=60)		$\chi 2$ p value
	No	%	No	%	
Pre test					
Mild	9	13.33	8	13.33	0.005
Moderate	51	86.67	52	86.67	0.576NS
Post test					
No depression	4	6.67	0	0	0.519
Mild	7	11.67	8	13.33	0.026*S
Moderate	49	81.66	52	86.67	

S-Significant, NS Non Significant,*p<.05

Table 4.3.6 presents the comparison of pre-test depression level among adolescent girls in the experimental group II and control group. 9 (15%) in the experimental group II and 8 (13.33%) adolescent girls in the control group had mild depression. Majority of the adolescent girls 51 (85%) in experimental group II and 52 (86.67%) adolescent girls in the control group had moderate level of depression. The groups had no significant difference as shown by chi-square value of 0.005 with p value of 0.576 between experimental group II and control group. Thus homogeneity between the groups is maintained.

Comparison of post-test depression level among adolescent girls in the experimental group II and control group reveals that 4 (6.67%) in the experimental group II had no depression after the intervention given. 7 (11.67%) in the experimental group II and 8 (13.33%) adolescent girls in the control group had mild depression. 49 (81.66 %) in the experimental group II and 52 (86.67%) adolescent girls in the control group had moderate level of depression. The samples between experimental group II and control group had significant difference as shown by chi square value of 0.519 with p value of <0.05. A significant statistical difference between the groups indicated that there is a significant reduction in the depression level in the experimental group II than the control group in the post-test.

Table 4.3.7: Comparison of level of depression among adolescent girls in the experimental group I and experimental group II during pre-test and post-test (n=120)

Level of depression	**Experimental group I (n=60)**		**Experimental group II (n=60)**		**$\chi 2$ p value**
	No	**%**	**No**	**%**	
Pre test					
Mild	8	13.33	9	13.33	1.629
Moderate	52	86.67	51	86.67	0.339NS

Table 4.3.7 Contd/

Level of depression	Experimental group I (n=60)		Experimental group II (n=60)		$\chi 2$ p value
	No	**%**	**No**	**%**	
Post test					
No	0	0	4	6.67	1.302
Mild	9	15	7	11.67	0.045*S
Moderate	51	85	49	81.66	

S-Significant, NS Non Significant,*p<.05

Table 4.3.7 presents the comparison of pre-test depression level among adolescent girls in the experimental group I and II. 8 (13.33%) adolescent girls in the experimental group I and 9 (15%) in the experimental group II had mild depression. Majority of the adolescent girls 52 (86.67%) in experimental group I and 51 (85%) adolescent girls in the experimental group II had moderate level of depression. The groups had no significant difference as shown by chi-square value of 1.629 with p value of 0.339. Thus homogeneity between the groups is maintained.

Comparison of post-test depression level among adolescent girls in the experimental group I and experimental group II reveals that 4 (6.67%) in the experimental group II had no depression after the intervention given. 9 (15%) adolescent girls in the experimental group I and 7 (11.67%) in the experimental group II had mild depression. 51 (85%) adolescent girls in the experimental group I and 49 (81.66%) in the experimental group II had moderate level of depression. The samples between experimental group I and experimental group II had significant difference as shown by chi square value of 1.302 with p value of <0.05. A significant statistical difference between the groups indicated that the reduction in the depression level was better with the experimental group II than the experimental group I in the post-test.

groups indicated that the reduction in the depression level was better with the experimental group II than the experimental group I in the post-test.

Table 4.3.8 : Comparison of level of depression among adolescent girls in the experimental group I, experimental group II and control group during pre test and post test (n=180)

Level of depression	Experimental group-I (n=60)		Experimental group II (n=60)		Control group (n=60)		$\chi2$ p value
	No	%	No	%	No	%	
Pre test							
Mild	8	13.33	9	13.33	8	13.33	0.093
Moderate	52	86.67	51	86.67	52	86.67	0.955NS
Post test							
No	0	0	4	6.67	0	0	8.653
Mild	9	15	7	11.67	8	13.33	0.049*S
Moderate	51	85	49	81.66	52	86.67	

S-Significant, NS Non Significant,*p<.05

Table 4.3.8 presents the comparison of pre-test depression level among adolescent girls in the experimental group I, experimental group II and control group. 8 (13.33%) adolescent girls each in the experimental group I and control group, and 9 (15%) in the experimental group II had mild depression. 52 (86.67%) adolescent girls each in the experimental group I and control group and 51 (85%) in experimental group II had moderate level of depression. The groups had no significant difference as shown by chi-square value of 0.093 with p value 0.955 between experimental group I, experimental group II and control group. Thus homogeneity between the groups is maintained.

Comparison of post-test depression level among adolescent girls reveals that 4 (6.67%) adolescent girls in the experimental group II had no depression after the intervention. 9 (15%) adolescent girls in the experimental group I, 7 (11.67%) in experimental group II and 8 (13.33%) in the control group had mild level of depression. 51(85%) adolescent girls in the experimental group I, 49 (81.66%) girls in the experimental group II and 52 (86.67%) in the control group had moderate depression. There is significant difference as shown by chi square value of 8.653 with p value< 0.05 between experimental group I, experimental group II and control group. A significant statistical difference between the groups indicated that there is a reduction in the depression level with the experimental group I and II than in control group.

Figure 4.3.4: Percentage distribution of level of depression among adolescent girls in the experimental group I during pre test and post test

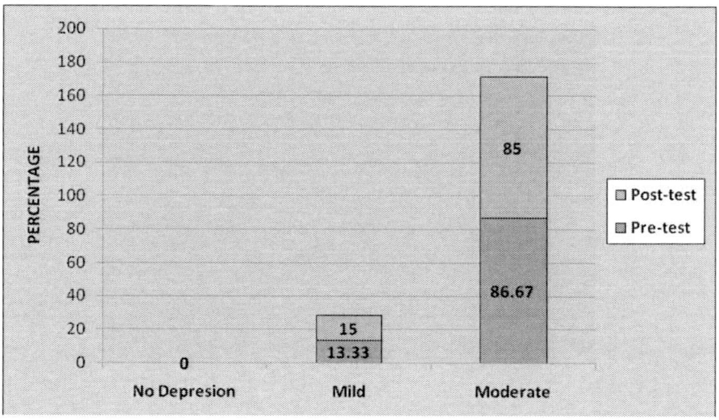

Figure 4.3.5: Percentage distribution of level of depression among adolescent girls in the experimental group II during pre-test and post-test.

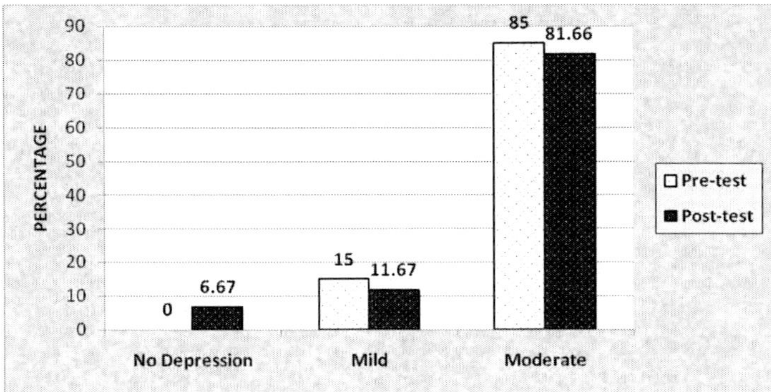

Figure 4.3.6: Percentage distribution of level of depression among adolescent girls in the control group during pre-test and post-test.

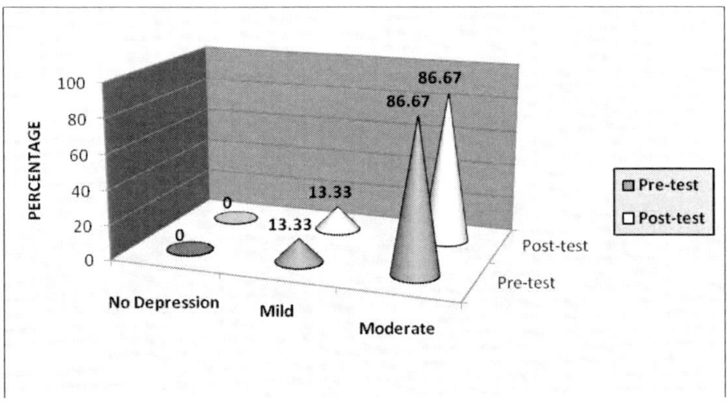

Table 4.3.9: Comparison of pre-test and post-test mean score of premenstrual syndrome among adolescent girls in the experimental group I (n=60)

Duration of study	Mean	SD	Mean Difference	Paired t value P value
Pre test	48.10	21.468	7.75	8.114
Post test	40.35	17.424		0.000***S

S-Significant, NS Non Significant,*p<.001**

Table 4.3.9 interprets that the adolescent girls pre-test level premenstrual syndrome was reduced from 48.10 mean score to 40.35 mean score during the post-test, which was highly significant at p <0.001. The comparison of mean score shows that the adolescent girls premenstrual syndrome was reduced between pre-test and post-test in experimental group I (7.75 Mean difference).

Table 4.3.10: Comparison of pre-test and post-test mean score of premenstrual syndrome among adolescent girls in the experimental group II (n=60)

Duration of study	Mean	SD	Mean Difference	Paired t value P value
Pre test	49.27	18.983	15.14	0.962
Post test	34.13	12.983		0.000***S

S-Significant, NS Non Significant, ***p<.001

Table 4.3.10 interprets that the adolescent girls pre-test level PMS was significantly reduced from 49.27 mean score to 34.13 mean score during the post-test which was highly significant at p <0.001. The comparison of mean score shows that the adolescent girls PMS was significantly reduced from pre-test to post-test in experimental group II (15.14 Mean difference).

Table 4.3.11: Comparison of pre-test and post-test mean score of premenstrual syndrome among adolescent girls in the control group (n=60)

Duration of study	Mean	SD	Mean Difference	Paired t value P value
Pre test	45.08	20.247	-4.403	-8.260
Post test	49.48	20.847		0.000***S

S-Significant, NS Non Significant, ***p<.001

Table 4.3.11 shows in the control group adolescent girls premenstrual syndrome was slightly increased from 45.08 mean score to 49.48 during the post- test at the level of p <0.001. The comparison of mean difference shows that the adolescent girls premenstrual syndrome was increased from pre-test to post-test in control group (-4.403 Mean difference).

Table 4.3.12: Comparison of pre-test and post-test mean score of depression among adolescent girls in the experimental group I (n=60)

Duration of study	Mean	SD	Mean Difference	Paired t value P value
Pre test	5.85	1.582	0.233	4.238
Post test	5.62	1.718		0.000***S

S-Significant, NS Non Significant, ***p<.001

Table 4.3.12 interprets that pre-test level depression of the adolescent girls in the experimental group I was reduced from the mean score 5.85 to 5.62 during the post-test. The comparison of mean score shows that there was a minimal reduction in the mean score of depression from pre-test to post-test which was minimally significant at p <0.001 (0.233 Mean difference).

Table 4.3.13: Comparison of pre-test and post-test mean score of depression among adolescent girls in the experimental group II (n=60)

Duration of study	Mean	SD	Mean Difference	Paired t value P value
Pre test	5.95	1.489	0.900	10.230
Post test	5.05	1.770		0.000***S

S-Significant, NS Non Significant, ***p<.001

Table 4.3.13 interprets that pre-test level depression of the adolescent girls in the experimental group II was significantly reduced from the mean score of 5.95 to 5.05 during the post test. Comparison of pre-test - post-test shows that the mean value of depression in post-test was lower than the pre-test which was highly significant at p <0.001 (Mean difference 0.900).

Table 4.3.14: Comparison of pre-test and post-test mean score of depression among adolescent girls in the control group (n=60)

Duration of study	Mean	SD	Mean Difference	Paired t value P value
Pre test	6.13	1.420	0.06	1.657
Post test	6.07	1.388		0.103NS

S-Significant, NS Non Significant

Table 4.3.14 highlights in the control group adolescent girls mean score depression was slightly decreased from 6.13 mean score to 6.07 during the post test. The comparison of mean score shows that there was a minimal reduction in the mean score of depression from pre-test to post-test . (Mean difference 0.06).

Table 4.3.15: Comparison of pre-test and post-test mean score of premenstrual syndrome among adolescent girls between the experimental group I and control group (n=120)

Duration of study	Experimental group I (n = 60)		Control group (n = 60)		Mean difference	Independent 't' value P value
	Mean	**SD**	**Mean**	**SD**		
Pre test	48.10	21.468	45.08	20.247	3.02	0.792 0.430NS
Post test	40.35	17.424	49.483	20.847	-9.133	-2.604 0.010*S

S-Significant, NS Non Significant, *p<.01

Table 4.3.15 depicts that the pre-test premenstrual syndrome mean score was 48.10 with SD 21.468 for the experimental group I and 45.08 with SD 20.247 for the control group and the independent t test value was 0.792 which was statistically not significant. No difference existed between the groups.

In post-test the premenstrual syndrome mean score was 40.35 with SD 17.424 in the experimental group I and 49.483 with SD 20.847 in the control group, and independent t test value was -2.604, a highly significant reduction in the premenstrual syndrome was noted among experimental group I than the control group at $p<0.05$.

Table 4.3.16 : Comparison of pre-test and post-test mean score of premenstrual syndrome among adolescent girls between the experimental groupII and control group (n=120)

Duration of study	Experimental group II (n = 60)		Control group (n = 60)		Mean difference	Independent 't' value P value
	Mean	**SD**	**Mean**	**SD**		
Pre test	49.27	18.983	45.08	20.247	4.19	1.168 0.245NS
Post test	34.13	12.983	49.48	20.847	-15.353	-17.720 0.000***S

S-Significant, NS Non Significant, ***p<.001

Table 4.3.16 depicts that the pre-test premenstrual syndrome mean score was 49.27 with SD 18.983 for the experimental group II and mean score of 45.08 with SD 20.247 for the control group and independent t test value was 1.168 which was statistically not significant. No difference existed between the groups.

In post-test the premenstrual syndrome mean score was 34.13 with SD 12.983 in the experimental group II and 49.48 with SD 20.847 in the control group, a highly significant reduction in the premenstrual syndrome was noted among experimental group II than the control group at $p<0.001$.

Table 4.3.17 : Comparison of pre-test and post-test mean score of premenstrual syndrome among adolescent girls between the experimental group I and experimental group II (n=120)

Duration of study	Experimental group I(n = 60)		Experimental group II (n =60)		Mean difference	Independent 't' value P value
	Mean	**SD**	**Mean**	**SD**		
Pre test	48.10	21.468	49.27	18.983	-1.17	-0.315 0.753NS
Post test	40.35	17.424	34.13	12.983	6.22	2.197 0.032*S

S Significant, NS Non Significant,*p<.05

Table 4.3.17 depicts that the pre-test premenstrual syndrome mean score was 48.10 with SD 21.468 for the experimental group I and 49.27 with SD 18.983 for the experimental group II and independent t test value was -.315, which was statistically not significant. No difference existed between the groups. In post-test the premenstrual syndrome mean score was 40.35 with SD 17.424 in the experimental group I and 34.13 with SD 12.983 in the experimental group II, a highly significant reduction in the premenstrual syndrome was noted among experimental group II than the experimental group I at $p<0.05$.

Figure 4.3.7: Comparison of pre-test and post-test mean score of premenstrual syndrome among adolescent girls between the experimental group I, II and control group

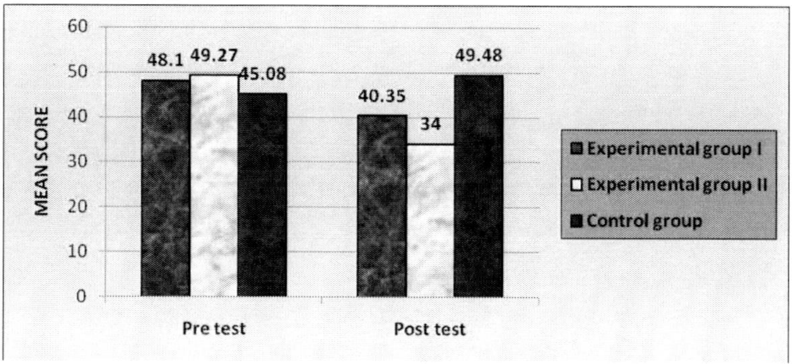

Table 4.3.18: Comparison of pre-test and post-test mean score of depression among adolescent girls between the experimental group I and control group (n=120)

Duration of study	Experimental group I (n = 60)		Control group (n =60)		Mean difference	Independent 't' value P value
	Mean	SD	Mean	SD		
Pre test	5.85	1.582	6.13	1.420	-0.28	-1.032 0.304NS
Post test	5.62	1.718	6.07	1.388	-0.45	-1.578 0.117NS

S-Significant, NS Non Significant

Table 4.3.18 presents that the pre-test depression mean score was 5.85 with SD 1.582 for the experimental group I and 6.13 with SD 1.420 for the control group and independent t test value was -1.032, which is statistically not significant. No difference existed between the groups. Comparison of post-test depression score between experimental group I and control group shows a minimal reduction from pre test to post test, but no significant statistical difference exists between the groups.

Table 4.3.19: Comparison of pre-test and post-test mean score of depression among adolescent girls between the experimental group II and control group (n=120)

Duration of study	Experimental group II (n=60)		Control group (n =60)		Mean difference	Independent 't' value P value
	Mean	**SD**	**Mean**	**SD**		
Pre test	5.95	1.489	6.13	1.420	-0.18	-0.690 0.491NS
Post test	5.05	1.770	6.07	1.388	-1.02	-3.501 0.001**S

S-Significant, NS Non Significant, **p<.01

Table 4.3.19 presents that the pre-test depression mean score was 5.95 with SD 1.489 for the experimental group II and 6.13 with SD 1.420 for the control group and independent t test value was -0.690, which is statistically not significant. No difference existed between the groups. Comparison of post-test depression score between experimental group II and control group shows a highly significant statistical difference existed at p<0.01 level.

Table 4.3.20: Comparison of pre-test and post-test mean score of depression among adolescent girls between the experimental group I and experimental group II (n=120)

Duration of study	Experimental group I (n =60)		Experimental group II (n =60)		Mean difference	Independent 't' value P value
	Mean	SD	Mean	SD		
Pre test	5.85	1.582	5.95	1.489	-0.1	-0.357 0.722NS
Post test	5.62	1.718	5.05	1.770	0.57	2.397 0.018*S

S-Significant, NS Non Significant,*p<.05

Table 4.3.20 presents that the pre-test depression mean score was 5.85 with SD 1.582 for the experimental group I and 5.95 with SD 1.489 for the experimental group II and independent t test value was -0.357, which is statistically not significant. Comparison of post-test depression score between experimental group I and experimental group II shows that a highly significant statistical difference existed at p< 0.05 level.

Figure 4.3.8: Comparison of pre-test and post-test mean score of depression among adolescent girls between the experimental group I, II and control group

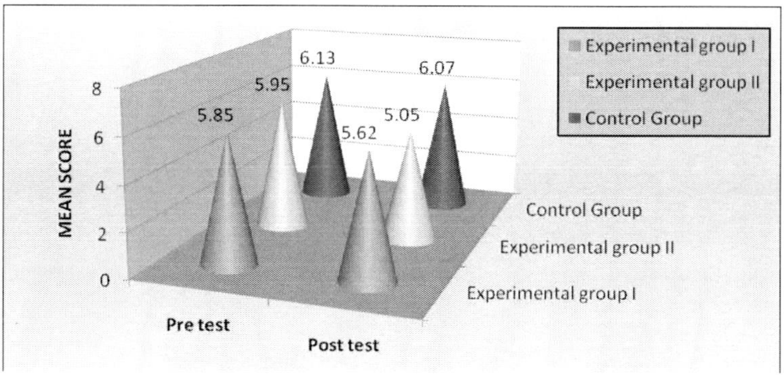

Table 4.3.21 : Comparison of pre-test mean score of premenstrual syndrome sub scale among adolescent girls between the experimental group I and control group (n=120)

Sub scale item	Experimental group I (n=60)		Control group (n=60)		Mean difference	Independent t t value p value
	Mean	**SD**	**Mean**	**SD**		
Pain	9.70	5.413	9.08	6.071	0.62	0.587 0.558 NS
Water retention	2.43	2.020	1.68	1.882	0.75	2.104 0.037*S
Autonomic reaction	4.97	3.737	3.60	3.136	1.37	2.170 0.032*S
Negative effect	11.43	6.578	9.93	6.772	1.5	1.231 0.221NS
Impaired concentration	4.80	4.524	6.88	6.272	-5.13	-4.882 0.000***S
Behavioural change	5.60	4.823	5.47	4.911	0.13	0.150 0.881NS
Arousal	7.20	4.679	6.02	4.862	1.18	1.358 0.177 NS
Control	1.973	575	2.42	4.288	-0.45	-0.624 0.534NS

S-Significant, NS Non Significant,*p<.05, ***p<.001

Table 4.3.21 indicates that there was significant statistical difference existed between the groups at p <.05 on water retention and autonomic reaction and at p <.001 on impaired concentration. No difference existed on other PMS sub scale such as pain, negative effect, behavioural change, arousal and control scores between the groups during pre test.

Table 4.3.22 : Comparison of pre-test mean score of premenstrual syndrome sub scale among adolescent girls between the experimental group II and control group (n=120)

Sub scale item	Experimental group II (n=60)		Control group (n=60)		Mean difference	Independent t value p value
	Mean	SD	Mean	SD		
Pain	9.80	5.908	9.08	6.071	0.72	0.655 0.514NS
Water retention	2.10	1.612	1.68	1.882	0.42	1.302 0.195NS
Autonomic reaction	5.35	3.621	3.60	3.136	1.75	2.830 0.005**S
Negative effect	10.10	6.025	9.93	6.772	0.17	1.142 0.887NS
Impaired concentration	5.47	4.036	6.88	6.772	-4.46	-4.389 0.000***S
Behavioural change	7.42	5.425	5.47	4.911	1.95	2.064 0.041*S
Arousal	7.42	4.893	6.02	4.862	1.4	1.572 0.119 NS
Control	1.62	2.624	2.42	4.288	-0.8	0.220 -1.233NS

S-Significant, NS Non Significant, *p<.05, **p<.01, ***p <.001

Table 4.3.22 indicates that there was highly significant statistical difference existed at p<.01 on autonomic reaction, at p < .001 on impaired concentration and at p <.05 on behavioural change and there was no significant difference existed on pain, water retention,negative effect, arousal and control between the groups on premenstrual syndrome sub scale score during pre-test.

Table 4.3.23 : Comparison of pre-test mean score of premenstrual syndrome sub scale among adolescent girls between the experimental group I and experimental group II (n=120)

Sub scale item	Experimental group I (n=60)		Experimental group II (n=60)		Mean difference	Independent t value p value
	Mean	SD	Mean	SD		
Pain	9.70	5.413	9.80	5.908	-0.1	-0.097 0.923 NS
Water retention	2.43	2.020	2.10	1.612	0.33	0.999 0.0320 NS
Autonomic reaction	4.97	3.737	5.35	3.621	-0.38	-0.571 0.569NS
Negative effect	11.43	6.578	10.10	6.025	1.33	1.158 0.249NS
Impaired concentration	4.80	4.524	5.47	4.036	0.764	-0.852 0.396 NS
Behavioural change	5.60	4.823	7.42	5.425	-1.82	-1.939 0.050*S
Arousal	7.20	4.679	7.42	4.893	-0.22	-0.248 0.805 NS
Control	1.973	575	1.62	2.624	0.35	-0.611 0.542 NS

S-Significant, NS Non Significant,*p<.05

Table 4.3.23 indicates that there was statistical difference existed between the experimental group I and experimental group II on premenstrualsyndrome sub scale score during pre-test at p <.05 on behavioural change and there was no significant difference existed on pain, water retention, autonomic reaction, negative effect, impaired concentration, arousal and control between the groups on premenstrual syndrome sub scale score during pre-test.

Table 4.3.24 : Comparison of post-test mean score of premenstrual syndrome sub scale among adolescent girls between the experimental group I and control group (n=120)

Sub scale item	Experimental group I (n=60)		Control group (n=60)		Mean difference	Independent t value p value
	Mean	**SD**	**Mean**	**SD**		
Pain	7.533	4.859	10.283	5.106	-2.750	-3.022 -0.003**S
Water retention	1.333	1.580	2.167	2.172	-0.834	-2.403 0.018*S
Autonomic reaction	4.216	3.537	5.667	3.587	-1.451	-2.229 0.028*S
Negative effect	9.85	6.832	11.75	6.08	-1.9	-1.609 0.110NS
Impaired concentration	4.766	4.204	7.3	5.264	-2.534	-2.913 0.004**S
Behavioural change	5.033	4.502	3.95	4.374	1.083	1.337 0.184NS
Arousal	5.783	5.415	7.433	5.419	-1.65	-1.668 0.098NS
Control	1.833	2.799	0.933	2.385	0.899	1.896 0.060NS

S-Significant, NS Non Significant,*p<.05, **p<.01

Table 4.3.24 highlights that there was highly significant statistical difference existed between the groups at p<0.05 on water retentionand autonomic reaction, at p <.01 on pain and impaired concentration. There was no significant difference existed on negative effect, behavioural change, arousal and control during post-test.

Table 4.3.25 : Comparison of post-test mean score of premenstrual syndrome sub scale among adolescent girls between the experimental group II and control group (n=120)

Sub scale item	Experimental group II (n=60)		Control group (n=60)		Mean difference	Independent t value p value
	Mean	SD	Mean	SD		
Pain	4.533	3.175	10.283	5.106	-5.75	-7.407 -0.000***S
Water retention	1.483	1.610	2.167	2.172	-0.683	-1.958 0.050*S
Autonomic reaction	4.20	3.058	5.667	3.587	-1.467	-2.410 0.017*S
Negative effect	6.93	3.922	11.75	6.08	-4.817	-5.156 0.000***S
Impaired concentration	4.65	3.531	7.3	5.264	-2.65	-3.239 0.002**S
Behavioural change	2.9	3.681	3.95	4.374	-1.05	-1.423 0.157NS
Arousal	8.733	5.909	7.433	5.419	3.314	1.256 0.212NS
Control	0.700	2.493	0.933	2.385	0.233	-0.524 0.601NS

S-Significant, NS Non Significant,*p<.05, **p<.01, ***p<.001

Table 4.3.25 highlights that there was highly significant statistical difference existed between the groups at p<0.05 on water retention and autonomic reaction, at p <.01 on impaired concentration, at p< .001 onpain and negative effect.There was no significant difference existed on behavioural change, arousal and control during post-test.

Table 4.3.26 : Comparison of post-test mean score of premenstrual syndrome sub scale among adolescent girls between the experimental group I and experimental group II (n=120)

Sub scale item	Experimental group I (n=60)		Experimental group II (n=60)		Mean difference	Independent t value p value
	Mean	**SD**	**Mean**	**SD**		
Pain	7.533	4.859	4.533	3.175	2.999	4.003 0.000***S
Water retention	1.333	1.580	1.483	1.610	0.150	-0.515 0.608NS
Autonomic reaction	4.216	3.537	4.20	3.058	0.016	0.028 0.978NS
Negative effect	9.85	6.832	6.933	3.922	2.917	2.868 0.005**S
Impaired concentration	4.766	4.204	4.650	3.531	0.116	0.165 0.870NS
Behavioural change	5.033	4.502	2.9	3.681	2.133	2.842 0.049*S
Arousal	5.783	5.415	8.733	5.909	-2.950	-2.851 0.005**S
Control	1.833	2.799	0.700	2.493	1.133	2.342 0.021*S

S-Significant, NS Non Significant,*p<.05, **p<.01, ***p<.001

Table 4.3.26 highlights that there was a highly significant statistical difference existed between the groups at p<0.05 on behavioural change and control, at p <.01 on negative effect and arousal, and at p <.001 on pain. There was no significant statistical difference existed between the groups on water retention, autonomic reaction, and impaired concentration.

Table 4.3.27: ANOVA of pre-test between experimental group I, II and control group for premenstrual syndrome and depression (n=180)

Variables	Experimental group I	Experimental group II	Control group	F value p value
	Pre-test mean	Pre-test mean	Pre-test mean	
PMS	48.10	49.27	45.08	0.681 0.507NS
Depression	5.85	5.95	6.13	0.552 0.577NS

S-Significant, NS Non Significant

From the ANOVA results in table 4.3.27it is evident that there was no significant difference between the groups as the F value shows 0.681 and 0.552 with p value 0.507 and 0.577 on premenstrual syndrome and depression. The ANOVA results further substantiate the't' test findings.

Table 4.3.28: ANOVA of post-test between experimental group I, II and control group for premenstrual syndrome and depression (n=180)

Variables	Experimental group I	Experimental group II	Control group	F value p value
	Post- test mean	Post- test mean	Post- test mean	
PMS	40.35	34.13	49.48	11.834 0.000***S
Depression	5.62	5.05	6.07	5.83 0.004**S

S-Significant, NS Non Significant, **p<.01, ***p<.001

From the ANOVA results in table 4.3.28 it is evident that there was a significant difference between the groups on premenstrual syndrome and depression as the F value shows 11.834 and 5.830 with p value <0.001 on

premenstrual syndrome and p<.01 on depression .The ANOVA results further substantiate the‘t’ test findings.

Table 4.3.29: ANOVA of pre-test, post-test between experimental group I, II and control group for premenstrual syndrome and depression (n=180)

Variables	Experimental group I		Experimental group II		Control group		F value p value
	Pre test mean	Post test mean	Pre test mean	Post test mean	Pre test mean	Post test mean	
PMS	48.10	40.35	49.27	34.13	45.08	49.48	2.633 0.043*S
Depression	5.85	5.62	5.95	5.05	6.13	6.07	4.466 0.012*S

S-Significant, NS Non Significant,*p<.05

From the ANOVA results in table 4.3.29 it is evident that there was a significant difference between the groups at p <0.05 on premenstrual syndrome and depression. The ANOVA results further substantiate the‘t’ test findings. Mean values of the three groups regarding premenstrual syndrome and depression revealed that the experimental group II values were more significant than other groups.

Section-4.4: Association of selected background variables with outcome variables of adolescent girls in the experimental group I, experimental group II and control group

Table 4.4.1: Association of selected background variables with post-test premenstrual syndrome among adolescent girls in the experimental group I (n=60)

Background variables	Level of premenstrual syndrome				$\chi 2$ p value
	Below median		Above median		
	No	%	No	%	
Age (in years)					
16-17	8	13.33	3	5	2.783
18-19	22	36.67	27	45	0.181NS
BMI					
Under weight	13	21.67	6	10	0.537
Normal	24	40	17	28.33	0.464NS
Class performance					
Good	18	30	14	23.33	1.071
Average	12	20	16	26.67	0.438 NS
Class missing					
Never	14	23.33	14	23.33	0.000
Yes	15	25	15	25	1.000NS
Always	1	1.67	1	1.67	
Age at menarche					
12-13 years	20	33.33	19	31.67	0.073
14-15 years	10	16.67	11	18.33	0.787NS
Menstrual duration					
1-2 days	1	1.67	1	1.67	5.613
3-4 days	11	18.33	20	33.33	0.050*S
5-6 days	18	30	9	15	
Menstrual interval					
15 – 20 days	2	3.33	1	1.67	1.857
21 – 25 days	10	16.67	9	15	0.603NS
26– 30 days	15	25	19	31.67	

31 – 35 days	3	5	1	1.67	

Table 4.4.1 Contd/-

Background variables	Level of premenstrual syndrome				χ2 p value
	Below median		Above median		
	No	%	No	%	
Menstrual flow					
Light	3	5	2	3.33	0.218
Medium	27	45	28	46.67	0.640NS
Menstrual regularity					
Yes	24	40	25	41.67	0.111
No	6	10	5	8.33	0.500NS

Significant, NS Non Significant,*p<.05

Table 4.4.1 portrays that there is a significant association existed for menstrual duration at $p < 0.05$ with premenstrual syndrome during post test among adolescent girls in the experimental group I

Table 4.4.2: Association of selected background variables with post-test premenstrual syndrome among adolescent girls in the experimental group II (n=60)

Background variables	Level of premenstrual syndrome				χ2 p value
	Below median		Above median		
	No	%	No	%	
Age (in years)					
16-17	6	10	6	10	1.021
18-19	24	40	24	40	0.600NS
BMI					
Under weight	17	28.33	22	36.67	1.832
Normal	13	21.67	8	13.33	0.279NS
Class performance					
Good	12	20	10	16.67	0.287
Average	18	30	20	13.33	0.789 NS
Class missing					
Never	17	28.33	17	28.33	0.000
Yes	13	21.67	13	21.67	1.000 NS

Table 4.4.2 Contd/-

Background variables	Level of premenstrual syndrome				χ2 p value
	Below median		Above median		
	No	%	No	%	
Age at menarche					
10-11 years	1	1.67	4	6.67	3.391
12-13 years	18	30	12	20	0.335NS
14-15 years	10	16.66	13	21.67	
>16 years	1	1.67	1	1.67	
Menstrual duration					
1-2 days	1	1.67	1	1.67	0.070
3-4 days	16	26.66	17	28.33	0.965NS
5-6 days	13	21.67	2	20	
Menstrual interval					
15 – 20 days	2	3.33	1	1.67	4.359
21 – 25 days	4	6.67	8	13.33	0.201NS
26– 30 days	19	31.67	20	33.33	
31 – 35 days	5	8.33	1	1.67	
Menstrual flow					
Light	6	10	1	1.67	5.281
Medium	20	33.33	27	45	0.048*S
Heavy	4	6.67	2	3.33	
Menstrual regularity					
Yes	24	40	29	48.33	4.043
No	6	10	1	1.67	0.049*S

Significant, NS Non Significant,*p<.05

Table 4.4.2 portrays that there is a significant association existed for menstrual regularity and menstrual flow at p <0.05with premenstrual syndrome during post test among adolescent girls in the experimental group II

Table 4.4.3: Association of selected background variables with post-test PMS among adolescent girls in the control group (n=60)

Background variables	Level of premenstrual syndrome				$\chi2$ p value
	Below median		Above median		
	No	%	No	%	
Age (in years)					
16-17	3	5	6	10	0.548
18-19	23	38.33	28	46.67	0.760NS
BMI					
Under weight	15	25	16	26.67	2.236
Normal	11	18.33	18	30	0.327NS
Class performance					
Good	14	23.33	23	38.34	1.291
Average	12	20	11	18.33	0.525NS
Class missing					
Never	18	30	17	28.33	2.564
Yes	8	13.34	17	28.33	0.278NS
Age at menarche					
10-11 years	2	3.33	5	8.33	5.520
12-13 years	16	26.67	19	31.67	0.238NS
14-15 years	8	13.33	10	16.67	
Menstrual duration					
1-2 days	13	21.67	17	28.33	0.070
3-4 days	13	21.67	17	28.33	0.965NS
Menstrual interval					
15 – 20 days	1	1.67	1	1.67	2.888
21 – 25 days	9	15	16	26.67	0.409NS
26– 30 days	15	25	13	21.66	
31 – 35 days	1	1.67	4	6.66	
Menstrual flow					
Light	2	3.33	5	8.33	5.577
Medium	23	38.34	21	35	0.233NS
Heavy	1	1.67	8	13.33	

Table 4.4.3 Contd/

Background variables	Level of premenstrual syndrome				$\chi2$ p value
	Below median		Above median		
	No	%	No	%	
Menstrual regularity					
Yes	22	36.67	27	45	1.901
No	4	6.67	7	11.67	0.387NS

S-Significant, NS Non Significant

Table 4.4.3 portrays no association existed for any of the variables with PMS during post test among adolescent girls in the control group.

Table 4.4.4: Association of selected background variables with post-test depression among adolescent girls in the experimental group I (n=60)

Background variables	Level of premenstrual syndrome				$\chi2$ p value
	Below median		Above median		
	No	%	No	%	
Age (in years)					
16-17	6	10	5	8.33	0.011
18-19	22	36.67	27	4.45	0.916NS
BMI					
Under weight	11	18.33	8	13.33	1.929
Normal	15	25	20	33.34	0.587NS
Over weight	1	1.67	3	5	
Obese	1	1.67	1	1.67	
Class performance					
Good	18	30	14	23.33	3.308
Average	10	16.67	18	30	0.129NS
Class missing					
Never	15	25	13	21.67	0.241
Yes	12	20	18	30	0.887NS

Always	1	1.67	1	1.67	

Table 4.4.4 Contd/-

Background variables	Level of premenstrual syndrome				$\chi2$ p value
	Below median		Above median		
	No	%	No	%	
Age at menarche					
10-11 years	2	3.33	1	1.67	1.124
12-13 years	15	25	21	35	0.771NS
14-15 years	10	16.67	9	15	
>16 years	1	1.67	1	1.67	
Menstrual duration					
1-2 days	1	1.67	2	3.33	1.607
3-4 days	12	20	18	30	0.448NS
5-6 days	15	25	12	20	
Menstrual flow					
Light	1	1.67	5	8.33	2.411
Medium	27	45	27	45	0.121NS
Menstrual interval					
15 – 20 days	1	1.67	3	5	3.042
21 – 25 days	8	13.33	10	16.66	0.385NS
26– 30 days	18	30	15	25	
31 – 35 days	1	1.67	4	6.67	
Menstrual regularity					
Yes	24	40	25	41.66	0.011
No	4	6.67	7	11.67	0.916NS

S-Significant, NS Non Significant

Table 4.4.4 portrays that there was no association existed for any of the variables with depression during post test among adolescent girls in the experimental group I.

Table 4.4.5: Association of selected background variables with post-test depression among adolescent girls in the experimental group II (n=60)

Background variables	Level of premenstrual syndrome				$\chi2$ p value
	Below median		Above median		
	No	%	No	%	
Age (in years)					
16-17	7	11.67	5	8.33	3.018
18-19	16	26.67	32	53.33	0.221NS
BMI					
Under weight	13	21.67	26	43.33	1.178
Normal	10	16.67	11	18.33	0.404NS
Class performance					
Good	15	25	7	11.67	13.092
Average	8	13.33	30	50	0.001**S
Class missing					
Never	17	28.33	17	28.3	
Yes	5	8.33	19	31.67	5.182
Always	1	1.67	1	1.67	0.075NS
Age at menarche					
10-11 years	1	1.67	3	5	5.693
12-13 years	8	13.33	23	38.33	0.128NS
14-15 years	13	21.67	10	16.66	
>16 years	1	1.67	1	1.67	
Menstrual duration					
1-2 days	1	1.67	1	1.67	0.501
3-4 days	11	18.33	21	35	0.778NS
5-6 days	11	18.33	15	25	
Menstrual interval					
15 – 20 days	2	3.33	1	1.67	1.209
21 – 25 days	4	6.67	8	13.33	0.751NS
26– 30 days	15	25	24	40	
31 – 35 days	2	3.33	4	6.67	

Background variables	Level of premenstrual syndrome				χ2 p value
	Below median		Above median		
	No	%	No	%	
Menstrual flow					
Light	2	3.33	5	8.33	0.433
Medium	19	31.67	28	46.67	0.805NS
Heavy	2	3.33	4	6.67	
Menstrual regularity					
Yes	21	35	32	53.34	0.319
No	2	3.33	5	8.33	0.697NS

S-Significant, NS Non Significant, **p<.01

Table 4.4.5 portrays that there is a significant association existed for class performance at p< 0.01 depression during post-test among adolescent girls in the experimental group II.

Table 4.4.6: Association of selected background variables with post-test depression among adolescent girls in the control group (n=60)

Background variables	Level of premenstrual syndrome				χ2 p value
	Below median		Above median		
	No	%	No	%	
Age (in years)					
16-17	5	8.33	4	6.67	0.336
18-19	23	38.33	28	46.67	0.562NS
BMI					
Under weight	16	26.67	15	25	1.630
Normal	12	20	17	28.33	0.427 NS
Class performance					

Good	19	31.67	18	30	0.851
Average	9	15	14	23.33	0.356NS

Table 4.4.6 Contd/

Background variables	Level of premenstrual syndrome				χ2 p value
	Below median		Above median		
	No	%	No	%	
Class missing					
Never	16	26.67	19	31.67	0.031
Yes	12	20	13	21.67	0.861NS
Age at menarche					
10-11 years	6	10	1	1.67	4.949
12-13 years	14	23.33	21	35	0.480NS
14-15 years	8	13.33	10	16.66	
Menstrual duration					
1-2 days	12	20	18	30	1.071
3-4 days	16	26.67	14	23.33	0.301NS
Menstrual interval					
15 – 20 days	1	1.67	1	1.67	1.586
21 – 25 days	14	23.33	11	18.33	0.663NS
26– 30 days	11	18.33	17	28.34	
31 – 35 days	2	3.33	3	5	
Menstrual flow					
Light	3	5	4	6.67	0.079
Medium	21	35	23	38.33	0.961NS
Heavy	4	6.67	5	8.33	
Menstrual regularity					
Yes	24	40	25	41.67	0.574
No	4	6.67	7	11.67	0.448NS

S-Significant NS Non Significant

Table 4.4.6 portrays that there is no significant association existed for any of the variables with depression during post test among adolescent girls in the control group.

Section- 4.5: Regression of selected outcome variables with selected background variables among adolescent girls in the experimental group I, II and control group

Table 4.5.1: Multiple Linear Regressions Analysis of post premenstrual syndrome with selected background variables of adolescent girls in the experimental group I (n=60)

Background Variables	Coefficient	Beta coefficient	't' value	'p' value	95% confidence interval
Constant					
BMI	0.025	0.006	0.043	0.966	-1.164--1.215
Class performance	-4.576	-.132	-.991	.326	-13.841--4.688
Class missing	1.113	.036	.279	.781	-6.892--9.117
Menstrual regularity	1.458	-0.033	-.244	.808	-13.446-10.531
Menstrual interval	.302	.061	.429	.669	-1.111--1.716
Menstrual duration	4.979	-321	-2.41	.019*S	-9.122--.835
Menstrual flow	-17.749	.-374	-2.79	.007**S	-30.515--4.983
Model summary -	**R2 value19.6%**				
Adjusted R square	**0.088**				

S Significant, NS Non Significant,*p<.05, **p<.01

Table 4.5.1 depicts an estimated 19.6% of variance of the background variables can be accounted for the linear combination ofpredictors, BMI, class performance class missing, menstrual regularity, menstrual interval, menstrual duration and menstrual flow. Menstrual duration and menstrual flow were most strongly related to premenstrual syndrome. Slopes for, BMI, class missing, and menstrual interval were positive andslopes for class performance, menstrual regularity, menstrual duration and menstrual flow were negative.slopes for class performance, menstrual regularity, menstrual duration and menstrual flow were negative.

Table 4.5.2: Multiple Linear Regressions Analysis of Post-test premenstrual syndrome with selected background variables of adolescent girls in the experimental group II (n=60)

Background Variables	Coefficient	Beta coefficient	't' value	'p' value	95%confidence interval
(Constant)					
BMI	-.527	-.088	-.650	.519	--2.156 -- 1.101
Class performance	.256	.010	.072	.943	6.865 --7.377
Class missing	-6.307	-.260	-1.962	.050*S	-12.758 -- .144
Menstrual regularity	-1.997	-.050	-.326	.746	-14.284 --10.290
Menstrual interval	-1.295	-.348	-2.274	.027*S	-2.438 ---.152
Menstrual duration	.160	.013	.094	.925	-3.246 --3.565
Menstrual flow	-7.982	-.288	-2.002	.049*S	-15.985 --.020
Model summary - R2 value		**20.9%**			
Adjusted R square 0.103					

S Significant, NS Non Significant, *p<.05

Table 4.5.2 depicts that the linear combination of the seven background variables had small linear relationship to the post premenstrual syndrome among adolescent girls in the experimental group II. R squared =0.209, adjusted R square = 0.103. An estimated 20.9% of variance of the background variables can be accounted for the linear combination of predictors, BMI, class performance, class missing, menstrual regularity, menstrual interval, menstrual duration and menstrual flow. Class missing, menstrual interval and menstrual flow were most strongly related to premenstrual syndrome. Slopes for class performance and menstrual duration were positive and slopes for BMI, class missing, menstrual interval,menstrual regularity and menstrual flow were negative.

Table 4.5.3: Multiple Linear Regressions Analysis of post-test premenstrual syndrome with selected background variables of adolescent girls in the control group (n=60)

Background Variables	Coefficient	Beta coefficient	't' value	'p' value	95% confidence interval
(Constant)					
BMI	1.197	.162	1.155	.253	-5.016 -19.124
Class performance	7.223	.170	1.204	.234	-15.847 -8.447
Class missing	-2.105	-.050	-.340	.735	-15.381 - 15.044
Menstrual regularity	1.199	.022	.157	.876	-13.446 --10.531
Menstrual interval	-.422	-.068	-.472	.639	-2.044 -1.511
Menstrual duration	-.438	-.021	-.147	.884	-6.824 -5.105
Menstrual flow	-6.784	-.169	-1.223	.227	-17.965 -4.361
Model summary - R2 value			**8.7%**		
Adjusted R square			**-.036**		

S Significant, NS Non Significant

Table 4.5.3 projects that the linear combination of the seven background variables had moderate linear relationship to the post premenstrual syndrome among adolescent girls in the control group.An estimated 8.7% of variance of the background variables can be accounted for the linear combination of predictors, BMI, class performance,class missing,menstrual regularity, menstrual interval, menstrual duration and menstrual flow. As indicated in table none of the variables were related to premenstrual syndrome with the control group. Slopes for BMI, class performance, and menstrual regularity were positive and slopes for class missing, menstrual interval, menstrual duration and menstrual flow were negative.

Table 4.5.4: Multiple Linear Regressions Analysis of post-test depression with selected background variables of adolescent girls in the experimental group 1 (n=60)

Background Variables	Coefficient	Beta coefficient	't' value	'p' value	95% confidence interval
(Constant)					
BMI	0.364	0.157	1.022	0.312	-.077--178
Class performance	-1.722	-0.090	-0.621	0.538	-1.269 --.715
Class missing	-0.030	-0.002	-0.013	0.990	-.885 --829
Menstrual regularity	-0.596	-0.024	-0.166	0.869	-1.284 --1.284
Menstrual interval	0.011	0.004	0.026	0.979	-.144 --.159
Menstrual duration	-0.872	-0.102	-00703	0.485	-.676 --.212
Menstrual flow	0.443	0.017	0.116	0.908	-1.313 --1.422
Model summary - R2 value		**5.1%**			
Adjusted R square -0.077					

S Significant, NS Non Significant

Table 4.5.4 depicts that the linear combination of the seven background variables had small linear relationship to the post-depression among adolescent girls in the experimental group I. An estimated 5.1% of variance of the background variables can be accounted for the linear combination of predictors, BMI, class performance, class missing, menstrual regularity, menstrual interval, menstrual duration and menstrual flow. As the table indicated no variables were related to post depression with experimental group I. Slopes for BMI, menstrual interval and menstrual flow were positive and slopes for class performance, class missing, menstrual regularity and menstrual duration were negative.

Table 4.5.5: Multiple Linear Regressions Analysis of post-test depression with selected background variables of adolescent girls in the experimental group II (n=60)

Background Variables	Coefficient	Beta coefficient	't' value	'p' value	95% confidence interval
(Constant)					
BMI	.007	.009	.062	.951	-.223 --.237
Class performance	-1.111	-.305	-2.22	.031*S	-2.15 ---.106
Class missing	-.715	-.216	-1.58	.121	-1.626 --.195
Menstrual regularity	.424	.078	.490	.626	-1.31 --2.157
Menstrual interval	-.032	-.063	-.395	.695	-.193 --.130
Menstrual duration	.231	.138	.963	.340	-.25 --.711
Menstrual flow	.723	.192	1.286	.204	-.406 --1.853
Model Summary-R2 value 15.3%					
Adjusted R Square				**0.039**	

S Significant NS Non Significant.*p < 0.05

Table 4.5.5 depicts that the linear combination of the seven background variables had small linear relationship to the post-depression among adolescent girls in the experimental group II. An estimated 15.3% of variance of the background variables can be accounted for the linear combination of predictors, BMI, class performance, class missing, menstrual regularity, menstrual interval, menstrual duration and menstrual flow. Class performance, were most strongly related to depression. Slopes for BMI, menstrual regularity, menstrual duration and menstrual flow were positive and slopes for class performance, class missing and menstrual interval were negative.

Table 4.5.6: Multiple Linear Regressions Analysis of post-depression with selected background variables of adolescent girls in the control group (n=60)

Background Variables	Coefficient	Beta coefficient	't' value	'p' value	95% confidence interval
(Constant)					
BMI	0.100	0.034	0.252	0.802	-.119 --.150
Class performance	-5.897	-0.350	-2.578	0.013*S	-1.647 ---.093
Class missing	4.254	0.256	1.802	0.077	-.044 --1.559
Menstrual regularity	-1.859	-0.088	-0.637	0.527	-1.452 --.529
Menstrual interval	0.025	0.010	0.075	0.941	-.114 --.117
Menstrual duration	-0.587	-0.072	-0.516	0.608	-.468 --.306
Menstrual flow	-0.287	-0.018	-0.136	0.893	-.731 --.705
Model Summary-R2 value15.2%					
Adjusted R Square 0.038					

S Significant NS Non Significant, *p <0.05

Table 4.5.6 depicts that the linear combination of the seven background variables had small linear relationship to the post-depression among adolescent girls in the control group. An estimated 15.2% of variance of the background variables can be accounted for the linear combination of predictors, BMI, class performance, class missing, menstrual regularity, menstrual interval, menstrual duration and menstrual flow. Class performance, were most strongly related to depression. Slopes for BMI, class missing and menstrual interval were positive and slopes for classperformance, menstrual regularity, menstrual duration and menstrual flow were negative.

CHAPTER V
DISCUSSION

Menstruation is a normal physiologic process for all women. It is normally a common experience throughout a woman's procreative period, and up to 90% account observing one or more symptoms during the days before menstruation. It isapproximated that as many as 3 of every 4 menstruating women have experienced some form of premenstrual syndrome. As this is a major problem disturbing a large number of female adolescent populations, the investigator is concentrating on premenstrual syndrome for her study. Many studies suggest that premenstrual discomfort is the main reason of frequent short term school absenteeism among adolescent girls. The aim of this study was to explore complementary and alternative therapies like foot reflexology and hot foot bath used by adolescent girls to minimize PMS.

The effect of alternative and complimentary therapy on pain reduction is less apparent. Many of the Indian studies could not be traced by the investigator in this area which might be due to lack of clear data from Indian women regarding the important aspects of women's life. This necessitates an in depth investigation and assessment of PMS. Hence the researcher felt the need to find the prevalence of premenstrual syndrome symptoms and other premenstrual discomforts among adolescent girls and the role of foot reflexology and hot foot bath as a basis to develop positive attitude to deal with premenstrual syndrome and depression in reduction of these symptoms. This study was done to find out the effectiveness of foot reflexology and hot foot bath on premenstrual syndrome among adolescent girls based on the objectives of the study. Strengths and limitations of the study were also provided.

5.1 Characteristics of the study samples

Adolescent girls with mild, moderate or strong premenstrual syndrome and mild or moderate depression were selected for the study. The adolescent girls who had severe premenstrual syndrome and severe depression were excluded from the study as the study intervention is focusing on preventive and promotive aspects.

5.1.1 Demographic variables

Descriptive analysis of the demographic variables (Table 4.2.1) indicated that 11 (18.33%) in the experimental group I, 12 (20%) in the experimental group II and 9 (15%) in the control group were belongs to the age group of 16-17 years. Majority of them, 49 (81.67%) in the experimental group I, 48 (80%) in the experimental group II and 51 (85%) in the control group were in the age group of 18-19 years. Regarding the class of studying 33 (55%) in the experimental group I, 22 (36.67%) in the experimental group II and 31 (51.67%) in the control group were studying in first year bachelor degree course. 27 (45%) in the experimental group I, 38 (63.33%) in the experimental group II and 29 (48.33%) in the control group were in the 2nd year bachelor degree classes.

Regarding the educational status of the fathers, 5 (8.33%) in the experimental group I, and 1 (1.67%) in the experimental group II and 2 (3.33%) in the control group had primary education. 14 (23.33%) in the experimental group I, 26 (43.33%) in the experimental group II and 20 (33.33%) in the control group had completed their high school education.19 (31.67%) in the experimental group I, 12 (20%) in the experimental group II

and 18 (30%) in the control group had completed their higher secondary education. 16 (26.67%), 17 (28.33%) and 19 (31.67 %) in the experimental group I, experimental group II and the control group were graduates respectively. 6 (10%) in the experimental group I, 4 (6.67%) in the experimental group II and 1 (1.67%) in the control group had completed their post-graduation degree.

With respect to educational status of the mother 3 (5%) in the experimental group I, 1 (1.67%) in the experimental group II and 3 (5%) in the control group had completed primary education. 15 (25%) in the experimental group I, 23 (38.33%) in the experimental group II and 22 (36.66%) in the control group completed high school education. 20 (33.33%), in the experimental group I, 16 (26.67%) each in the experimental groupII and control group were completed higher secondary education. 18 (30%) in the experimental group I, 17 (28.33%) in the experimental group II and 16 (26.67%) in the control group were graduates. 4 (6.67%) in the experimental group I, 3 (5%) each in the experimental group II and control group were post graduates.

Regarding the occupation of fathers 3(5%) in the experimental group I, 5 (8.33%) in the experimental group II and 1 (1.67%) in control group were unemployed. 11 (18.33%) in the experimental group I and 4 (6.67%) in the experimental group II , 9 (15%) in the control group were unskilled workers. 10 (16.67%) in the experimental group I and 16 (26.67%) in the experimental group II, 11 (18.33%) in the control group were skilled workers. Majority of them 36 (60%), 35 (58.33%), 39 (65%) in the experimental group I, II and control group were professionals respectively. Regarding the occupation of mothers majority of them 43(71.67%), 52(86.67%), 48(80%) in the

experimental group I, II and control group were house wives respectively. 3(5%) in the experimental group I, 1(1.67%) in the experimental group II and 2 (3.33%)in the control group were skilled workers.14(23.33%) in the experimental group I,7(11.67%) in the experimental group II and 10 (16.67%) in the control group were professionals.

The total family income per month highlighted that11 (18.33%) each in the experimental group I and control group and 20(33.33%) in the experimental group II had family income range of Rs. <2500-2500. 5 (8.33%) in the experimental group I, 4(6.67%) in the experimental group II and 7 (11.66%) in the control group had a family income range of Rs 2501- 5000 per month. This signified that nearly half of the adolescent girls were from lower middle class family. 6 (10%) in the experimental groupI,12 (20%) in the experimental group II and 5 (8.33%) in the control group had a family income range of Rs. 5001-7500.19 (31.67%) in the experimental group I, 12 (20%) in the experimental group II and 22(36.67%) in the control group had a family income range of Rs 7501-10000.19 (31.67%) in the experimental group I and 12 (20%) in the experimental group II and 15 (25%) in the control group had a family income range of Rs >10000. The chi square revealed homogeneity between the experimental group I, II and the control group with regard to all the demographic variables except for place of residence where a dispersion at $p < 0.05$ was noted between the groups.

5.1.2 Personal variables

Distribution of personal variables indicated that (Table 4.2.2) majority of the adolescent girls 41(68.33%) in the experimental group I, 39 (65%) in the experimental group II and 29 (48.33%) in the control group had

normal weight. 19(31.67%) in the experimental group I, 21 (35%) in the experimental group II and 31 (51.67%) in the control group had underweight. The class performance of adolescent girls revealed that 32 (53.33%) in the experimental group I, 22(36.67%) in the experimental group II and 37(61.67%) in the control group were having good performance.28 (46.67%) in the experimental group I, 38(63.33%) in the experimental group II and 23 (38.33%) in the control group were having fair performance in the class.

Regarding the class absenteeism 28 (46.67%) in the experimental group I, 34 (56.66%) each in the experimental group II and control group had never missed their classes during menstruation. 30(50%) in the experimental group I, 25 (41.66%) each in the experimental group II and the control group had missed their classes during menstruation.2 (3.33%) in the experimental group I and 1(1.67%) each in the experimental group II and control group were always missing their classes during menstruation. Exam missing of the adolescent girls during menstruation revealed that 11(18.33%) in the experimental group I, 6(10%) in the experimental group II and 13 (21.67%) in the control group were missing exams during menstruation and remaining girls were not missing their classes during menstruation.13(21.67%) adolescent girls in the experimental group I, 18 (30%) in the experimental group II and 20 (33.33%) in the control group were using some or other remedial measures to control premenstrual syndrome symptoms. The chi square revealed homogeneity between the experimental group I, II and the control group with regard to all the personal variables except for BMI and class performance where dispersion at $p < 0.05$ was noted between the groups.

5.1.3 Gynaecologic variables

Distribution of gynaecological variables among adolescent girls (Table 4.2.3) showed that 2 (3.33%) in the experimental group I and 4 (6.67%) in the experimental group II and 7(11.67%) in the control group had attained menarche at the age of 10-11 years. Majority of them, 37 (61.67%) adolescent girls in the experimental group I, 31(51.67%) in the experimental group II and 35 (58.33%) in the control group attained menarche at 12-13 years. 20(33.33%) in the experimental group I, 23 (38.34%) in the experimental group II and 17 (28.33%) in the control group adolescent girls had attained menarche at 14-15 years. 1 (1.67%) each in the experimental group I and control group and 2 (3.33%) in the experimental group II attained menarche after > 16 years of age.

With regard to menstrual duration, 2 (3.33%) girls in the experimental group I and 1(1.67%) each in the experimental group II and control group had menstrual bleeding for 1-2 days. Majority of the girls, 31(51.67%), 33(55%), and 30(50%) adolescent girls had menstrual bleeding for 3-4 days in experimental group I,II and control group respectively. 27(45%) in the experimental group I, 26(43.33%) in the experimental group II and 29(48.33%) in the control group had menstrual bleeding for 5-6 days. Regarding menstrual regularity majority of the adolescent girls 49(81.67%) each in experimental group I and control group and 53 (88.33%) in experimental group II had regular menstrual cycle.Remaining girls were having irregularity in menstruation.

With regard to menstrual interval 3(5%) adolescent girls each in the experimental group I and II and 1 (1.67%) in the control group had menstrual

interval of 15-20 days. 19 (31.67%) in the experimental group I, 12 (20%) in the experimental group II and 26 (43.33%) in control group had menstrualinterval of 21-25 days. 34(56.66%) in experimental group I, 39 (65%) in experimental group II and 28(46.67%) in control group had menstrual interval of 26-30 days.4 (6.67%) in experimental group I, 6(10%) in the experimental group II and 5(8.33%) in the control group had menstrual interval of 31-35 days.

4(6.67%) in experimental group I, 7 (11.67%) each in the experimental group II and control group had light menstrual flow. Most of them, 52 (86.66%) in experimental group I, 47 (78.33%) in the experimental group II and 44(73.33%) in control group had medium menstrual flow. 4 (6.67%) in experimental group I, 6 (10%) in experimental group II and 9 (15%) in control group had heavy menstrual blood flow. PMS awareness highlighted that majority of adolescent girls 27 (45%) in experimental group I, 36 (60%) in experimental group II and 28 (46.67%) in the control group were aware about premenstrual syndrome. The remaining girls were unaware of premenstrual syndrome. The chi square revealed no significant dispersion between experimental groups I, II and the control group with regard to all the gynaecological variables.

5.2 Prevalence of premenstrual syndrome and depression

The first objective of the study was to determine the prevalence of premenstrual syndrome and depression among adolescent girls

In this study, the prevalence of PMS was 70% as measured by Moos Menstrual distress questionnaire. This is in agreement with Sunita Kumari and Ankur Sachdeva (2016) reported that the prevalence of PMS was 70-90%. Similarly prevalence rate of PMS was 78.5% in a study conducted

byManal Ahmad Al-Batanony and Sultan Fahad AL-Nohair (2014). In Sri Lanka among a sample of adolescents Chandraratne and Gunawardena (2011) had reported 65.7% PMS. Similarly a cross-sectional survey of 1295 rural adolescent girls aged 13-19 years in Malaysia by Wong showed that most participants (63.1%) identified as having PMS.

In the present study prevalence of depression was 52.6%. These findings were in consistent with the findings of the study by Bakhshani, Mousavi and Khodabandeh (2009) among young Iranian women stated that 72.3% samples were having depression associated with PMS. Similarly a study done by Padmavathi, Srinivasagam, Raja Sankarand Kokilavani (2014) the prevalence of depression associated with premenstrual syndrome was found to be 60%.Findings by KeshavJee, Mary Pushpa Bara and Ajay Kumar Bakhla (2017) supported the findings of the current study. They had found out that 30-76% of women with premenstrual dysphoric disorder had history of depression.

5.3 Effectiveness of foot reflexology on PMS and depression

The second objective of the study is to determine the effect of foot reflexology on premenstrual syndrome and depression

This study showed (Table 4.3.1) that in the pretest 22 (36.67%) adolescent girls in the experimental group I had mild PMS. 36 (60%) adolescent girls had moderate PMS and strong premenstrual syndrome was found among 2 (3.33%) adolescent girls in the experimental group I. These findings are in consistent with the findings of the study of Hetal Jain and Avani Parekh, (2015) done among married and unmarried females in Charusat, Changa, India and which has stated that 63% of the subjects had

mild to moderate symptoms of PMS. Similarly Sharma, Malhotarc, Taneja, and Saha (2010) studied the type and frequency of the problems related to menstruation among adolescent girls in New Delhi, India. The results revealed that 63.1% had one or other symptoms of premenstrual syndrome. In this study the post-test premenstrual syndrome level among adolescent girls in the experimental group I revealed 39 (65%) adolescent girls had mild PMS, 19 (31.67%) adolescent girls had moderate PMS and strong premenstrual syndrome was found among 2 (3.33%) adolescent girls in the experimental group I. There is a reduction in the premenstrual syndrome level in the post test when compared to pre-test.

Assessment of premenstrual syndrome (Table 4.3.9) among adolescent girls in the experimental group I showed significant reduction in the mean score from 48.10 during pretest to 40.35 during the post-test. Comparison of the pretest-post-test showed that the mean value of premenstrual syndrome in the post test was lower (mean= 40.35, SD=17.424) than the pre- test (mean= 48.10, SD=21.468) and the paired t value is 8.114 in the experimental group I, which was highly significant at $p < 0.001$. The study findings were consistent with the results of other researchers. Study conducted by Edith Meszaros Crowand Emilien Jeannot (2017) on dualistic treatment approach to premenstrual syndrome among general female population found that in post-test, 22% samples got moderate relief from premenstrual syndrome.

When assessing depression (Table 4.3.12) among adolescent girls in the experimental group I showed significant reduction in mean score from 5.85 during the pretest to 5.62 during the post-test. Comparison of the pretest post-test shows that the mean value of depression in the post test was lower (mean= 5.62, SD=1.718) than the pre- test (mean= 5.85, SD=1.582) in the

experimental group I, and the paired t value showed 4.238 which was highly significant at $p < 0.001$. It is in consistent with the study of Mozhgan Soheili, Fatemeh Nazari, Vahid Shaygannejad and Mahboobeh Valiani (2017) after performing reflexology and relaxation interventions for 4 weeks, twice weekly for 40 minutes reported significant reduction in the severity of anxiety, stress and depression among multiple sclerosis patients.

5.4 Effectiveness of hot foot bath on PMS and depression

The third objective of the study is to determine the effectiveness of hot foot bath on premenstrual syndrome and depression

This study showed (Table 4.3.2) 19 (31.67%) adolescent girls had mild PMS, 38 (63.34%) had moderate PMS and strong premenstrual syndrome was found among 2 (3.33%) adolescent girls in the experimental group II. Whereas the post-test PMS level revealed 55 (91.67%) adolescent girls had mild PMS and 5 (8.33%) had moderate PMS. The study results showed a significant reduction in the premenstrual syndrome level in the post test when compared to pre-test.

Assessment of premenstrual syndrome (Table 4.3.10) among adolescent girls in the experimental group II showed significant reduction in the mean score from 49.27 during the pretest to 34.13 during the post-test. Comparison of the pretest posttest showed that the mean value of premenstrual syndrome in the post test was lower (mean= 34.13, SD=12.983) than the pre- test (mean= 49.27, SD=18.983) in the experimental group II, which was highly significant at $p < 0.001$. The present study is supported by the research conducted by Yang, Chen, Lee,Fang and Chao (2010) where they reported a significant reduction in fatigue and improvement in sleep quality after hot foot bath therapy among gynaecologic cancer patients. Findings of the study by Hadayat Amasha, Ragaa Ali Mohamed and Haylaa Nageeb (2015) came in agreement with the findings of the present study. They reported that most of the study subjects (87%) used CAT like hydrotherapy minimized the symptoms of premenstrual syndrome. Findings of Marwa Mohamed, Asmaa Bandrawy, and Amir Gabr (2016) supported the study findings of the current study. They found the mean value ±SD of daily symptoms report score for group before starting the treatment was (49.09± 3.85), while it was decreased to (34.37 ±4.07) after the end of the treatment, representing a highly significant decrease (P<0.001)after the treatment program.

When assessing depression (Table 4.3.13) among adolescent girls in the experimental group II showed significant reduction in the mean score from 5.95 during the pretest to 5.05 during the post-test. Comparison of the pretest- posttest showed that the mean value of depression in the post test was lower (mean= 5.05, SD=1.770) than the pretest (mean= 5.95, SD=1.489) in the experimental group II, and the paired t value showed 10.23 which was highly significant at p <0.001. This result was confirmed by that of Mooventhan and Nivethitha (2014) who conducted a study to investigate the scientific evidence-based effects of hydrotherapy on various systems of the body and found significant reduction in tension, fatigue, memory, mood and negative state points after warm bath therapy.

5.5 Compare the effect of foot reflexology on premenstrual syndrome(PMS) and depression with control group.

The fourth objective of the study is to compare the effect of foot reflexology on PMS and depression with control group.

The pre-test premenstrual syndrome (Table 4.3.15) mean score was 48.10 with SD 21.468 for the experimental group I and 45.08 with SD 20.247 for the control group and the independent t test value was 0.792 which was statistically not significant. No difference existed between the groups during pre-test. In post-test the premenstrual syndrome mean score was 40.35 with SD 17.424 in the experimental group I and 49.483 with SD 20.847 in the control group, and independent t test value was -2.604, a highly significant reduction in the premenstrual syndrome was noted among experimental group I than the control group at $p<0.01$. Comparison of premenstrual syndrome mean difference in the post test between experimental group I and control group (9.133 mean difference) shows that the adolescent girls premenstrual syndrome had reduced in the experimental group I after foot reflexology technique at the level of $p<0.01$. Regarding improvement in PMS symptoms the result was supported by Sareh et al., (2013) who said that foot reflexology is effective in improvement of physical and mental symptoms of PMS. Similarly Lee et al. (2012) reported a reduction in premenstrual syndrome and dysmenorrhea and improvement in the temperature of lower abdomen with reflexology which was similar to the findings of the present study. There was also a significant reduction existed between the experimental group I and control group on premenstrual syndrome sub scale score (Table 4.3.24) during post-test at $p<.05$ on water retention andautonomic reaction, pain and impaired concentration at $p<.01$. The present study indicated that there was a statistically significant difference in the premenstrual syndrome between the

groups during post-test. **Hence the first hypothesis of the study (H1) "There is a significant difference in premenstrual syndrome among adolescent girls who receive foot reflexology than who do not" was accepted by the researcher.**

The pre-test depression mean score (Table 4.3.18) was 5.85 with SD 1.582 for the experimental group I and 6.13 with SD 1.42 for the control group and independent t test value was - 1.032, which is statistically not significant. No difference existed between the groups. Comparison of post-test depression score between experimental group I and control group shows a minimal reduction from pre-test to post test in both the groups, and independent t test value was -1.578 which is statistically not significant. **Hence the second hypothesis (H2) "There is a significant difference in depression among adolescent girls who receive foot reflexology than who do not" was rejected by the researcher.** In the literature review no studies indicating the effectiveness of reflexology on depression levels of adolescent girls with premenstrual syndrome were found. However there are studies examining the effectiveness of reflexology on depression in different sample population. In a study by Eom et.al (2008) performed in 47 women with an average age of 78.5 years, the geriatric depression scale was applied to the women before and after a reflexology application. Significant decreases in depressive symptoms were found after reflexology therapy. Study findings of Aydin, Aslan and Yalcin (2016) is in agreement with the present study. In their study to determine the effect of reflexology on the level of depression in women with over active bladder,they found out that foot reflexology relieved urinary and depressive symptoms and had a positive effect on quality of life. Similarly the present study findings were consistent with the findings of the study done by Yun-Mi Lee (2005) in identifying the effects of a foot

reflexology massage on depression and stress responses reported that there was a statistically significant difference in depression and perceived stress after giving foot reflexology therapy for 6 weeks.

5.6 Compare the effect of hot foot bath therapy on premenstrual syndrome with control group

The fifth objective of the study is to compare the effect of hot foot bath therapy on premenstrual syndrome with control group.

The present study depicts that (Table 4.3.16) the pre-test premenstrual syndrome mean score was 49.27 with SD 18.983 for the experimental group II and mean score of 45.08 with SD 20.247 for the control group and independent t test value was 1.168 which was statistically not significant. No difference existed between the groups during pre-test. In the post-test the premenstrual syndrome mean score was 34.13 with SD 12.983 in the experimental group II and 49.48 with SD 20.847 in the control group, and independent t test value was -17.720 which shows a highly significant reduction in the premenstrual syndrome among experimental group II than the control group at $p<0.001$ during post-test. Comparison of premenstrual syndrome mean difference in the post test between experimental group II and control group (-15.353 mean difference) shows that the adolescent girls premenstrual syndrome had reduced in the experimental group II after hot foot bath therapy at the level of $p <0.001$. There was also a reduction in the experimental group II premenstrual syndrome sub scale(Table 4.3.25) scores on water retention and autonomic reaction at $p<.05$, at $p<.01$ on impaired concentration and at $p < .001$ on pain and negative effect after hot foot bath therapy. The present study is supported by the research conducted by Yang,Chen,Lee,Fang and Chao (2010) where they reported a significant reduction

in fatigue and improvement in sleep quality after hot foot bath therapy among gynecologic cancer patients. The present study indicated that there were statistically significant differences in the premenstrual syndrome between the groups during post-test. **Hence the third hypothesis of the study (H3) "There is a significant difference in premenstrual syndrome among adolescent girls who receive hot foot bath therapy than who do not" was accepted by the researcher.**

In the present study (Table 4.3.19) the pre-test depression mean score was 5.95 with SD 1.489 for the experimental group II and 6.13 with SD 1.420 for the control group and independent t test value was -0.690, which was statistically not significant. No difference existed between groups during pre-test. Comparison of post-test depression score between experimental group II (mean 5.05, SD 1.770) and control group (mean 6.07, SD 1.388) and the independent t test value was -3.501 reveals a highly significant statistical difference at $p < 0.001$ level. **Hence the fourth hypothesis (H4) "There is a significant difference in depression among adolescent girls who receive hot foot bath therapy than who do not" was accepted by the researcher.**

Hot foot bath therapy on premenstrual syndrome and depression has not been researched sufficiently (may be subjected for correction). Though there are no similar studies found enough evidences are available on the effect
of hot foot therapy in various other disorders. The positive findings of the present study are consistent with the assumption that hot foot bath therapy is beneficial among adolescent girls with premenstrual syndrome and depression.

5.7 Compare the effect of foot reflexology vs. hot foot bath on premenstrual syndrome and depression

The sixth objective of the study is to compare the effect of foot reflexology vs. hot foot bath on premenstrual syndrome and depression

The pre-test premenstrual syndrome mean score (Table 4.3.17) was 48.10 with SD 21.468 for the experimental group I and 49.27 with SD 18.983 for the experimental group II and independent t test value was -0.315, which was statistically not significant. No difference existed between the groups during pre-test. In post-test the premenstrual syndrome mean score was 40.35 with SD 17.424 in the experimental group I and 34.13

with SD 12.983 in the experimental group II, and the independent t test value was 2.197, a highly significant reduction in the premenstrual syndrome was noted among experimental group II than the experimental group I at $p<0.05$.

Comparison of premenstrual syndrome post-test mean score in experimental group I and II reveals that the adolescent girls post- test mean score of premenstrual syndrome in experimental group II had significantly reduced from 34.13 to post-test mean score of 40.35 in experimental group I, which was highly significant at $p<0.05$ and comparison of mean difference shows that the adolescent girls premenstrual syndrome had reduced more in experimental group II (15.14mean difference) with hot foot bath therapy than in experimental group I (7.75 mean difference) with foot reflexology. The present study is in agreement with the study conducted by Naseri, Rahmani, Nerir, Salari and Moshkani Farahani (2016) in identifying the effects of foot reflexology and foot bath on modifying sleep in patients with acute coronary syndrome, the result revealed that the difference between foot bath group and the control group was more than that of the reflexology and

control group in the inter group evaluations in terms of decreased sleep disturbance, supplementary sleep average and sleep efficacy. There was also a highly significant statistical difference existed on premenstrual syndrome sub scale score between the groups at $p<0.05$ on behavioural change and control, at $p<.01$ on negative effect and arousal and at $p<.001$ on pain.Similarly in the control group there was a significant increase in the mean score of premenstrual syndrome from 45.08 to 49.483 at the level of $p<0.001$ (Negative significance), when compared to the pretest -posttest.**Hence the hypothesis (H5) "There is a significant difference in premenstrual syndrome among adolescent girls who receive hot foot bath therapy than who receive foot reflexology" was accepted by the researcher.**

The pre-test depression mean score (Table 4.3.20) was 5.85 with SD 1.582 for the experimental group I and 5.95 with SD 1.489 for the experimental group II and independent t test value was -0.357, which is statistically not significant. No difference existed between the groups during pre-test. Comparison of post-test depression score between experimental group I (mean 5.62, SD 1.718) and experimental group II (mean 5.05, SD 1.770) shows that a highly significant statistical difference existed at $p< 0.05$ level. The adolescent girls in the experimental group I and II reported less depression, three months after the foot reflexology and hot foot bath therapy implementation, while no significant changes were found in the control group. Comparison of mean difference shows that the adolescent girlsdepression had reduced more in experimental group II than in experimental group I. **Hence the hypothesis (H6) "There is a significant difference in depression among adolescent girls who receive hot foot bath therapy than who receive foot reflexology was accepted by the researcher.**

From the ANOVA results in table4.3.29 it is evident that there was a significant difference between the groups at $p<0.05$ on premenstrual syndrome and depression. The ANOVA results further substantiate the't' test findings. Mean values of the three groups regarding premenstrual syndrome and depression revealed that the experimental group II values are more significant than other groups.

5.8 Association of background variables with outcome variables

The seventh objective of the study is to find the association between selected demographic variables (age, BMI, place of residence, age at menarche, class performance, class missing during menstruation, menstrual duration, menstrual interval and menstrual flow) with post premenstrual syndrome and depression among adolescent girls.

The association between selected background variables with premenstrual syndrome in the experimental group I, II and the control group was determined through Chi square test. A significant association existed for menstrual duration at $p < 0.05$ with post- test premenstrual syndrome among adolescent girls in the experimental group I (Table 4.4.1). A significant association existed for menstrual flow and menstrual regularity at $p < 0.05$ with post-test premenstrual syndrome among adolescent girls in the experimental group II (Table 4.4.2). The study findings were consistent with the results of other researchers. Ray, Mishra, Roy and Das (2010) reported a significant association of menstrual regularity with premenstrual syndrome in their study conducted at West Bengal among the urban and rural adolescent girls. Association existed between the post test depression and class performance at $p < 0.001$ in the experimental group II(Table 4.4.5).

This result was further substantiated by the multiple linear regressions. Table 4.5.1 projected that the linear combination of the seven background variables (BMI, class performance, class missing,menstrual regularity, menstrual interval, menstrual duration and menstrual flow) had small linear relationship to the post premenstrual syndrome, among adolescent girls in the experimental group I, R squared =0.196, adjusted R square = .088.An estimated 19.6% of variance of the background variables can be accounted for the linear combination of predictors, BMI, class performance, class missing,menstrual regularity, menstrual interval, menstrual duration and menstrual flow. Menstrual duration and menstrual flow were most strongly related to premenstrual syndrome. Slopes for, BMI, class missing, and menstrual interval were positive and slopes for class performance, menstrual regularity, menstrual duration and menstrual flow were negative.

Table 4.5.2 depicts that the linear combination of the seven background variables had small linear relationship to the post premenstrual syndrome among adolescent girls in the experimental group II, R squared =0.209, adjusted R square = 0.103. An estimated 20.9% of variance of the background variables can be accounted for the linear combination of predictors, BMI, class performance, class missing, menstrual regularity, menstrual interval, menstrual duration and menstrual flow. Class missing, menstrual interval and menstrual flow were most strongly related to premenstrual syndrome. Slopes for class performance and menstrual duration were positive and slopes for, BMI, class missing, menstrual regularity, menstrual interval and menstrual flow were negative.

The subjects who underwent complementary and alternative therapies like foot reflexology and hot foot bath felt that they have learnt a

skill that can be used for relaxation and in stressful situations. They experienced that these therapies helped in decreasing tensions, depression, premenstrual symptoms, illness and other bodily disorders. They felt happy, satisfied, cheerful and light hearted. Furthermore, they experienced a complete well-being in their body. In this present study, physical and psychological improvement in subjects with PMS, after the implementation of CAT appears to have the potential to generate positive effects on complete well being. This discussion concludes that foot reflexology and hot foot bath could be used as nursing intervention for adolescent girls with PMS in the outpatient and inpatient units of various hospitals, community centers, schools and in the community at large by nursing staff, community health nurses, school health nurses and student nurses. This intervention could be enforced even for normal adolescent girls and who is in pre pubertal phase as well as to the women in general.

5.9 Strengths of the study

- This study was a prospective randomized controlled trial design.
- Simple random sampling technique was used to allot the samples in to the experimental groups and the control group
- The foot reflex therapy intervention was delivered on one to one basis by the investigator and the investigator underwent professional training on foot reflexology.
- Hot foot bath therapy was delivered to the samples by the investigator herself

- The basic techniques of foot reflex therapy and hot foot bath was taught to the adolescent girls with appropriate illustrations
- Foot reflexology and hot foot bath therapy leaflet was issued to the samples free of cost

- Continuity of care was reinforced by the investigator
- A low rate of refusal and absence of attrition is an evidence for the feasibility of delivering the intervention and its acceptability to the adolescent girls
- The control group adolescent girls were also taught foot reflexology and hot foot bath therapy after completion of the study
- The adolescent girls of both the groups expressed the usefulness of these therapies
- Prospective daily record was used in this study
- Included theory based skill intervention
- Allowed to interact freely regarding reproductive health issues
- The duration and pattern of practice used for the study was an added advantage
- Most participants said that they felt incredibly relaxed after completing the therapies

5.10 Limitations of the study

- The study was limited to college adolescent girls of bachelor degree course, which is not guidance to other adolescent girls.
- To monitor prospective daily record, daily symptom dairy was used as the assessment tool. The instrument has 47 premenstrual syndrome symptoms, and the too many number of the item to record in daily symptom dairy seemed to be very difficult for the participants
- Participants were limited to 1st and 2nd year bachelor degree students so it could not be representative of adolescent age which included only 17 to 19 years old.
- Measurement of psychological phenomena is complex and difficult

CHAPTER VI

SUMMARY, CONCLUSIONS, IMPLICATIONS AND RECOMMENDATIONS

6.1 SUMMARY

Premenstrual syndrome (PMS) is a very common condition that affects a woman's emotions, physical health, and behaviour during certain days of the menstrual cycle, generally just before her menstruation. It start during the week before menstruation and alleviate when the menstruation flow begin. 85% of the menstruating women are affected with its symptoms and it interferes with some aspect of women's life such as daily routine at work, home, social activity or relationships, which even change their conduct and well being and can affect their family, social and work circle.

As many as 50%-60% of women with severe PMS have an underlying psychiatric disorder mainly depression. The occurrence of premenstrual syndrome is according to ICD-10 criteria, nearly 42% of women experience mild PMS and 31.7% experience moderate PMS (Samia Tabassum, 2005). Approximately 5% of women experience severe premenstrual symptoms mainly depression, anxiety, irritability and loss of confidence, and physical symptoms like bloating and mastalgia. Premenstrual symptoms are a common problem among the adolescent girls.PMS symptoms adversely affects the academic and social performances of the students and emotional well being and it has got a negative impact on the quality of life of adolescent girls.The prevalence rate of PMS was more among adolescent girls and if we are not treating it properly may lead to poor academic performance and severe mental problems.So there is a terribe need

to teach and learn different nursing strategies which is cost effective and harmless to them. As the premenstrual syndrome and depression can be managed by life style modification and stress management, the researcher wanted to apply nursing strategies inclusive of stress management through alternative and complementary therapies such as foot reflexology and hot foot bath therapy among adolescent girls.

The objectives of the study were to:

- ❖ Determine the prevalence of premenstrual syndrome and depression among adolescent girls
- ❖ Determine the effectiveness of foot reflexology on premenstrual syndrome and depression
- ❖ Determine the effectiveness of hot foot bath on premenstrual syndrome and depression
- ❖ Compare the effect of foot reflexology on PMS and depression with control group.
- ❖ Compare the effect of hot foot bath therapy on PMS and depression with control group.
- ❖ Compare the effect of foot reflexology vs. hot foot bath on PMS and depression
- ❖ Find the association between selected demographic variables with post premenstrual syndrome and depression. (age, BMI, place of residence, age at menarche, class performance, class missing during menstruation, menstrual duration, menstrual interval, menstrual flow).

The formulated study hypotheses were:

- ❖ **H_1:** There is a significant difference in premenstrual syndrome among adolescent girls who receive foot reflexology than who do not.

- **H_2:** There is a significant difference in depression among adolescent girls who receive foot reflexology than who do not.
- **H_3:** There is a significant difference in premenstrual syndrome among adolescent girls who receive hot foot bath therapy than who do not.
- **H_4:** There is a significant difference in depression among adolescent girls who receive hot foot bath therapy than who do not.
- **H_5:** There is a significant difference in premenstrual syndrome among adolescent girls who receive hot foot bath therapy than who receive foot reflexology.
- **H_6:** There is a significant difference in depression among adolescent girls who receive hot foot bath therapy than who receive foot reflexology.

Related literature were reviewed and grouped under various aspects. The review of literature enabled the investigator to formulate the conceptual framework, to construct questionnaire, to determine the methodology of the study and plan for the data analysis in an effective way. Conceptual framework was based on Nola J. Pender's Health Promotion Model. The major concept of this model is individual characteristics and experiences, behaviour specific cognitions and behaviour specific outcome. The adolescent girls awareness on premenstrual syndrome and depression and the knowledge of foot reflexology and hot foot bath therapy could help to plan a strategy which leads to implementation of health promoting behaviour such as relieving of PMS and depression.

Research methodology

It is a true experimental study. This quantitative research used a pretest posttest control group design with arts and science colleges as the unit of randomization. Manipulation included the foot reflexology technique to experimental group I and hot foot bath therapy to experimental group II. There were a total of 12 sessions each in both groups and weekly one session and each session lasted for 15 minutes. Foot reflexology techniques were implemented by the researcher to the experimental group I. A total of 6 groups with 10 adolescent girls in each group were grouped for foot reflexology session. This was done once in a week 15 minutes for 3 months in the college hostel during evening time after the college hours. Hot foot bath therapy was given by the researcher to the experimental group II. A total of 6 groups with 10 adolescent girls in each group were grouped for hot foot bath therapy session. This was done once in a week 15 minutes for 3 months in the college hostel during morning time before the college hours.The control group adolescent girls were asked to continue with their normal routine activities and researcher completed the assessments at the same time intervals as that of the experimental groups.

The study was conducted in selected arts and science colleges at Pathanamthitta district, colleges were assigned randomly to experimental and control group using simple random sampling technique (lottery method) and the population included adolescent girls with mild, moderate or strong PMS along with mild or moderate depression and those who fulfilled the inclusion criteria during the period of study were selected as samples. Estimated sample size was 180 with 60 subjects in each group.

Description of research Tools: The tool was prepared based on the objectives of the study. The data collection tool consisted of

Part I: Background variables:

Section -A: Demographic variables

Section -B: Personal variables

Section -C: Gynaecological variables

Part II: Standardized Menstrual Distress Questionnaire.

The tool was constructed by Rudolf. H. Moos to assess the premenstrual syndrome symptoms among adolescent girls.The questionnaire contains description of symptoms classified in to eight categories (total 47 items) such as, Pain (6) concentration (9)behavioural change (5) autonomic reaction (4) water retention (4) negative effect (8) arousal (5) and control (6).

Part III: IPAT Depression Scale (Personal Assessment Inventory Scale)

The tool was constructed by Samuel E. Krug and James E. Laughlin. It contains 40 statements about how people feel or think at one time or other.

Part IV: Daily Symptom Dairy

It is used to assess the prospective record of premenstrual syndrome symptoms.

The instruments were validated by experts and reliability was checked using test-retest method. A pilot study was conducted with 20 samples in each group which helped to assess the reliability and feasibility of the instruments. Modifications were done based on the pilot study results and experts recommendations.

Data Collection procedure

The data were collected three times; during survey, pretest, and post test.

Survey phase

Simple random sampling technique was followed to select the colleges for the study. Data collection was done among 1st and 2nd year bachelor degree girls of six selected arts and science colleges to identify adolescent girls who fulfilled the inclusion criteria. Retrospective and prospective premenstrual symptoms were collected from the girls.

Data Collection phase

A total of 180 samples, (60 samples in each group) who were full filling the inclusion criteria were selected as study subjects for data collection.

Intervention phase

After the pretest, samples from experimental group I undergone foot reflexology for 15 minutes once a week for 3 months and experimental group II samples were undergone hot foot bath therapy for 15 minutes once a week for 3 months.Control group samples were asked to continue the routine activity.

Major findings of the study

Homogeneity was maintained in the background variables of all three groups except for place of residence in demographic variables and BMI and class performance under personal variables.

Prevalence of PMS and depression among adolescent girls

The prevalence of premenstrual syndrome and depression in the present study was done among 1097 samples. The study result showed that

36.37% samples were having mild PMS, 30.54% samples were having moderate PMS. 2.37% and 0.55% samples were having strong and severe PMS respectively. Prevalence of depression showed that 12.03% samples were having mild depression, 37.38% samples were having moderate depression and 2.19% samples were having severe depression.

Effect of foot reflexology on premenstrual syndrome and depression

The adolescent girls pre-test level premenstrual syndrome was reduced from 48.10 mean score to 40.35 mean score during the post-test, which was highly significant at $p < .05$. The comparison of mean difference showed that the adolescent girls premenstrual syndrome was reduced from pre-test to post-test in experimental group I (7.75 Mean Difference). The pre-test level depression of the adolescent girls in the experimental group I was reduced from the mean score of 5.85 to 5.62 during the post-test. The comparison of mean difference shows that there was a minimal reduction in the mean score of depression from pre-test to post-test which was minimally significant at p <.05 . (0.233 Mean Difference).

Effectiveness of hot foot bath on premenstrual syndrome and depression

The adolescent girls pre-test level premenstrual syndrome was significantly reduced from 49.27 mean score to 34.13 mean score during the post-test which was highly significant at p <0.001. The comparison of mean difference shows that the adolescent girls premenstrual syndrome was significantly reduced from pre-test to post-test in experimental group II (15.14 Mean Difference). The pre-test level depression of the adolescent girls in the experimental group II was significantly reduced from the mean score 5.95 to

5.05 during the post test. Comparison of pretest-posttest showed that the mean value of depression in post-test was lower than the pre-test which was highly significant at p <0.05. (Mean difference 0.900).

Comparison of foot reflexology on premenstrual syndrome with control group.

The pre test premenstrual syndrome mean score was 48.10 with the SD of 21.468 for the experimental group I and 45.08 with the SD of 20.247 for the control group and independent t- test value was 0.792 with p value 0.424 which was statistically not significant. No difference existed between the groups. In the post test premenstrual syndrome mean score was 40.35 with SD of 17.424 in the experimental group I and

49.483 with SD of 20.847 in the control group. A highly significant reduction in the premenstrual syndrome was noted in the experimental group I than the control group at $p < 0.01$. In the experimental group I, 65%, 31.67% and 3.33% samples had mild, moderate and strong premenstrual syndrome whereas in the control group 33.33%, 63.34% and 3.33 % had mild, moderate and strong premenstrual syndrome.There was also a highly significant statistical difference existed between the groups on premenstrual syndrome sub scale score for water retention and autonomic reaction at $p<.05$,pain and impaired concentration at $p <.01$ during post test.

Comparison of foot reflexology on depression with control group.

The pre-test depression mean score was 5.85 with SD 1.582 for the experimental group I and 6.13 with SD 1.42 for the control group and

Independent t test value was 1.032, which was statistically not significant. No difference existed between the groups. The post-test depressions mean score was 5.62 with SD 1.718 for the experimental group I and 6.07 with SD 1.388 for the control group and independent t test value was 1.578, which was statistically not significant. No difference existed between the groups. Comparison of post-test depression score between experimental group I and control group showed a minimal reduction from pre-test to post test, but no significant statistical difference existed between the groups.

Compare the effect of hot foot bath on premenstrual syndrome with control group.

The pre-test premenstrual syndrome mean score was 49.27 with the SD of 18.983 for the experimental group II and 45.08 with the SD of 20.247 for the control group and independent t- test value was 1.168 with p value 0.245 which was statistically not significant. No difference existed between the groups. In the post test premenstrual syndrome mean score was 34.13 with SD of 12.983 in the experimental group II and

49.483 with SD of 20.847 in the control group. A highly significant reduction in the premenstrual syndrome was noted in the experimental group II than the control group at p<0.001.In the experimental group II, 91.67% and 8.33% samples had mild and moderate premenstrual syndrome whereas in the control group 33.33%, 63.34% and 3.33% samples were having mild, moderate and strong premenstrual syndrome. There was a highly significant statistical difference existed between the groups at p<0.05 on water retention and autonomic reaction,at p<.01 on impaired concentration, at p<.001 onpain and negative effect during post test.

Compare the effect of hot foot bath therapy on depression with control group.

The pre-test depression mean score was 5.95 with SD 1.489 for the experimental group II and 6.13 with SD 1.420 for the control group and independent t test value was 0.690, which was statistically not significant. No difference existed between the groups. The post test depression mean score was 5.05 with SD 1.770 for the experimental group II and 6.07 with SD 1.388 for the control group and independent t test value was 3.501, which was highly significant at p <0.001. A highly significant reduction in the depression was noted in the experimental group II than control group.

Compare the effect of foot reflexology vshot foot bath on premenstrual syndromeand depression

The pre-test premenstrual syndrome mean score was 48.10 with SD 21.468 for the experimental group I and 49.27 with SD 18.983 for the experimental group II and independent t test value was 0.315, which was statistically not significant. No difference existed between the groups. In post-test the premenstrual syndrome mean score was 40.35 with SD 17.424 in the experimental group I and 34.13 with SD 12.983 in the experimental group II, a highly significant reduction in the premenstrual syndrome was noted among experimental group II than the experimental group I at $p < 0.05$. There was a highly significant statistical difference existed between the groups at $p<0.05$ on behavioural change and control ,at $p <.01$ on negative effect and arousal, pain at $p <.001$ on premenstrual syndrome sub scale score during post test. The pre-test depression mean score was 5.85 with SD 1.582 for the experimental group I and 5.95 with SD 1.489 for the experimental group II

and independent t test value was 0.357, which was statistically not significant. The post-test depression mean score was 5.62 with SD 1.718 for the experimental group I and 5.05 with SD 2.397 for the experimental group II and independent t test value was 2.397. Comparison of post-test depression score between experimental group I and experimental group II showed that a highly significant statistical difference existed at $p< 0.05$ level.

From the ANOVA results it is evident that there was a significant difference between the groups at $p<0.05$ on premenstrual syndrome (F value 2.633 and p value 0.043) and at $p <.05$ on depression (F value 4.466 and p value 0.012).Mean values of the three groups regarding premenstrual syndrome and depression revealed that the experimental group II values were more significant than other groups and observed that the hot foot bath therapy was more effective than foot reflexology in reducing premenstrual syndrome and depression.

Association between selected demographic variables with premensyrual syndrome and depression

Significant association existed between menstrual duration at $p< 0.05$ with post test premenstrual syndrome among adolescent girls in the experimental group I. Significant association was shown between the post test premenstrual syndrome with menstrual flow and menstrual regularity at $p<0.05$ level among adolescent girls in the experimental group II and there was no significant association existed between post test premenstrual syndrome and demographic variables in the control group. Significant association was shown between the post test depression and class performance at $p < 0.001$ level among adolescent girls in the experimental

group II and there was no significant association existed between post test depression and demographic variables in the control group.

Regression analysis of post premenstrual syndrome with background variables indicated that menstrual duration and menstrual flow were the most powerful predictors in the experimental group I. Class missing,menstrual interval and menstrual flow were most strongly related to post premenstrual syndrome in experimental group II. Predictors for post depression were class performance in both experimental group II and in control group.

6.2 Conclusion

The study results indicated that the adolescent girls achieved an overall positive result from foot reflexology and hot foot bath therapy. The pre test assessment revealed that majority of the samples had mild to moderate premenstrual syndrome and mild to moderate depression. The premenstrual syndrome and depression experienced by the adolescent girls significantly reduced after foot reflexology and hot foot bath therapy.It is desirable to prepare adolescent girls with menstrual health and complementary and alternative medicine as a basis to develop skill and positive attitude to deal with premenstrual syndrome and depression.The result highlighted that these therapies were an effective technique in the reduction of PMS and depression.

Complementary and alternative therapies like foot reflexology and hot bath therapy can be implemented in the educational institutions, hospitals and community centres to create a change in the attitude and practice of adolescent girls regarding premenstrual syndrome and menstrual hygiene. Findings of this study were consistent with the other literature and supported

by studies conducted all around the world. Based on the selection of samples, sample size and support from other studies, the findings could be generalized to adolescent girls with premenstrual syndrome and depression.

6.3 Implications of the study

Some of the implications derived from the present study in various practice and educational settings of nursing are as follows

6.3.1 Nursing Practice

The present study shows that premenstrual syndrome and depression are very much predominant among adolescent girls at colleges. To reduce this trouble, nurses and midwives working in the urban and rural health centres should attempt various alternative and complementary therapies along with health information to the public. The study reveals that foot reflexology technique and hot foot bath therapy has an explicit impact in reducing premenstrual syndrome symptoms and depression. To extent its significance it is essential for the nurses and midwives to create awareness about these therapies among adolescent girls. Professional educational offerings could be provided by advanced practice nurses.

Recent life style of the adolescents causes so many stressful effects to the body which can be relieved by foot reflexology and hot foot bath therapy and it aid in improving the performance in our life day by day. Complementary therapies make adolescent girls emotional, physiological, and spiritual health improve and increase the value of their life. Itpropose high level of safety and effectiveness. Learning reflexology and hot foot bath therapy and its application are quite easy; there is no limitation for people to apply it at any time and anywhere. It also leads to many benefits in health concern such as it helps in easing day-to-day stresses. These alternative therapies can be integrated into clinic and home based models of health care to improve body health condition and well-being in terms of physical, emotional, and spiritual level of adolescent girls with PMS. These therapies are free from any drugs and chemical, and it is a wide option for many health problems and is well accepted by adolescent girls.

6.3.2 Nursing Education

Nurse educators are considering including complementary and alternative medicine in nursing curricula at least in part by the ever-increasing public enthusiasm for these therapies. Setting educational standards and developing consistent curricula for CAM therapies will help students emerge from academic programs prepared for safe and effective practice and with skills to assess the effectiveness and participate in the research of CAM therapies. This helps not only the public to achieve optimum health but also help individual students to modify their life style.

Nurses and midwives should be oriented on practice of effective complimentary therapies such as foot reflexology and hot foot bath therapy based on evidence based research through in-service and continuing nursing education courses. Nurse educators should provide sufficient opportunisms for their students to practice and extend the awareness of CAM therapies like foot reflexology and hot foot bath therapy because reflexology and hot foot bath are alternative therapies, which is cost effective and has no side effects, and improves emotional, physiological, and spiritual health which in turn increase the value of their life.

Nurse educators should train the Multi-purpose health workers on complementary and alternative medicine (CAM) practices as they are the grass root level primary care providers in the rural areas. This not only helpful to the adolescent girls and women in the community area but also helps to take care of themselves too. Since these therapies are easy to perform and cost effective methods it will be much beneficial to the rural people as the rural area people are not having adequate health care facility and many of them belongs to low financial background status.

Nursing curriculum in India already incorporated PMS concept from the year 2005. Indian nursing council can launch separate certificate program on complementary and alternative medicine practice as the public is more enthusiastic on these therapies and many rely upon these therapies for their various health conditions. In addition to the various use of complementary and alternative therapies by the public, other reasons for pursing the issue in nursing education include: media attention to the positive outcomes of complementary and alternative therapy (CAT), nursing interest and the increasing number of articles on the topic in highly respected professional journals, the inclusion of these therapies in medical curricula, the necessity to provide culturally congruent care, and increasing governmental legitimacy both nursing students and nursing faculty are likely to be among the millions of people who have turned to CAT for a wide variety of reasons.

6.3.3 Nursing administration

Nurse administrators/officers should formulate policies and protocols on complementary and alternative medicine practices with added evidence based research. Nurse administrators /officers should employ proper

integration of complementary and alternative medicine practices in managing various health related disorders at different levels of prevention and it could definitely improve patients' quality of life. Such management practices should be regulated as policies and protocols to make sure informed practice by all the health care team members.

Nurse administrators must make provision for educating their team members regarding CAM practices. Education can affect nurses' perceptions of their ability to provide evidence based care and thus their ability to empower their patients. Patient empowerment is a fundamental concept in nursing care and can be accomplished through trust, communication, education, support, and mutual goal setting. It helps to integrate a holistic approach to patient centered care. It could also help identify possible learning needs of nurses and may be beneficial to educators and managers alike. Nurse administrators with their capacity can disseminate through mass media the healing power and advantages of foot reflexology and hot foot bath therapy and other relevant CAM practices to the community. This would increase creativity, interest and motivation among the community members for a healthy living.

6.3.4 Nursing research

There are so many issues which nurses face in attempting to use research-based literature and when conducting research in the field of complementary therapies. In spite of the considerable interest among the nurses in using such therapies, there can be difficulties in gaining access to such literature and using it to inform practice. Rising standards of accountability create expectations for nurses on evidence based research and

on sources of information which inform safe and effective practice. In order to accomplish this there should be an adequate support, motivation and encouragement by the management and authorities of organization to conduct various research activities and this could be the mission of many novice nurses.

Indulging in research activities and motivating to do the research activities could improve the body of professional knowledge. Such new evidence based knowledge can improve the health status among adolescent girls. Incidence and prevalence of premenstrual syndrome can be studied through community survey research. Since there are very less research studies on effect of complementary and alternative therapies like foot reflexology and hot foot bath in reducing premenstrual syndrome among adolescent girls, it will be beneficial to conduct research on lived in experience of adolescent girls with premenstrual syndrome, relating to the demographic characteristics, foot reflexology technique, hot foot bath therapy and its effects and hindrances encountered by adolescent girls to have a better understanding of the problem.

6.4 Recommendations for further study

- The study should be replicated in other geographical locations to gain a more comprehensive understanding of adolescent girlsperceptions on complementary and alternative therapies and premenstrual syndrome.
- Studies may be replicated in other settings especially in community areas.
- The study can be replicated on larger samples
- A similar study can be conducted with the use of video assisted or computer assisted teaching

- Study can be done with use of latest mobile app to enforce regular treatment.
- The study can be replicated among adolescent girls of different age groups
- The study can be replicated among women in different occupations.
- Long term follow up studies for a period of 1-3 years can be conducted
- Complementary and alternative therapy practices can be extended to adolescent girls with dysmenorrhea and other menstrual problems
- More research could be conducted to explore more on complementary and alternative therapies

- Further exploration about the relationship between complementary and alternative therapies and premenstrual syndrome is necessary to know more about on this subject
- More research focusing on medical providers' perceptions of complementary and alternative therapy use and premenstrual syndrome would be helpful to promote teamwork and an interdisciplinary approach to strategic care.

Printed by BoD™in Norderstedt, Germany

9 781805 254218